DADsercise

Lose Weight! Build Muscle!
It's Child's Play

Perry Schnacker

authorHOUSE™

1663 LIBERTY DRIVE, SUITE 200
BLOOMINGTON, INDIANA 47403
(800) 839-8640
WWW.AUTHORHOUSE.COM

First published by AuthorHouse 09/14/05

ISBN: 1-4208-8022-5 (sc)

Library of Congress Control Number: 2005907814

Printed in the United States of America
Bloomington, Indiana

This book is printed on acid-free paper.

Notice:

The information in this book is not meant to replace proper exercise training. All forms of exercise pose inherent risk. Extra precautions are required when children are involved. Every exercise needs to be evaluated based on the adult's strength and ability as well as the child's strength and ability. If there is any risk or concern the exercise should not be performed. The author advises the readers to take full responsibility for their safety as well as their children's safety. You should get doctors approval for you and for your children before beginning this or any form of exercise.

I need to thank my wife for supporting me in all my crazy ideas. I couldn't have lost the weight and especially put this book together without her support.

I have to thank my children. They have been great. They were and still are very cooperative in helping me DADsercise. There would be no DADsercise without them.

Last, thanks to my brother Tracy for taking my writing and making it sound good. There is no way this would have gotten done without his help.

Table of Contents

Introduction – What started all this

As soon as my son Daniel, who was diagnosed with Down Syndrome, joined our family as our third child, his heart became the focus of our doctors. Knowing that many children with Down Syndrome are born with defects in the heart chambers, the doctors painstakingly took him through numerous tests to determine if a problem existed. Daniel was not an exception. *Our* hearts heavy but hopeful for the best, my wife and I scheduled the surgery designed to patch the holes. As a former wrestler and football player, I'm accustomed to taking on challenges head on, but I knew that to have a child go through open-heart surgery at five months would be an emotional event, its outcome life-changing.

When so many aspects of my life were in chaos and seemingly out of my hands, I began to concentrate on elements in my life that I could control. After some introspection I came to the realization that I was probably headed for heart problems myself. I was the heaviest I had ever been, packing 215 pounds on a 5' 7" frame. Even the thought of any meaningful exercise made me shudder. I would squeeze any health-conscious thought to the bottom of my priority list (if it even made the list). However, after a while the fear of my kids having to grow up without a father and my wife having to raise these three children by herself began to slowly burn a hole in my conscience.

It's not that I hadn't thought about my condition before this. I attacked the stairs from time to time instead of the elevator — the stairs usually won. After two or three flights I was working on catching my breath; after four flights I needed the oxygen masks to drop from the ceiling. When I finished wrestling or playing football with my kids, Pain and Soreness, like two smirking athletic trainers, would gingerly escort me off the playing field to the medicine cabinet. Angry at myself, I knew that I had allowed myself to not only lose a healthy lifestyle — I needed a compass and a map to find it. What I wanted, no, what I *needed* was to get in shape to enjoy an active and fulfilling life.

After Daniel's surgery and long convalescence, I resolved to make a common-sense diet and an exercise program a priority. I know, I know. You just saw the word "diet." If you're like me "diet" is a four-letter word. A diet to someone who was raised in Central Nebraska, meat and potato country, means hold the gravy on the taters. I knew that for me to go on any type of diet program would be like expecting a wolf to go vegetarian. It wasn't going to happen. So without seeking the advice of any consultants, diet regimens, or 900 numbers, I just decided to stop eating so many fatty foods, consume a few less calories, and start exercising. Getting through the first month was the most difficult, but once I started to see and feel the results, you couldn't stop me with a slab of ribs from reaching my goals.

I could tell you that my exuberance to reach my goals led me to start training for body building contests and marathons, but that would be dishonest. To be perfectly frank, my early experiences with running were not that enjoyable. My coaches, barking and growling at the heels of stragglers, would run my teammates and me until we knew that our lunch was going to be revisited. We always wondered if we had insulted them without our knowing it and were now being punished for it. In my youth it was hard to see the true benefits of exercise. Today, I have discovered that running can be enjoyable. Once I made the concession that exercise did not have to cause palpitations, I found that I really enjoyed taking in the vistas along the miles of pathways in my community. Everyone is different, however, and you or your doctor needs to determine how strenuous your exercise routine should be.

As my weight started falling gradually like leaves in October, I could feel my energy levels rising. It became easier to slide down to the floor to play with my kids who welcomed me to their space with surprised enthusiasm. Adam and Ellen loved their "new" dad who felt like he was sipping from the fountain of youth. This new vigor brought back some college memories when my buddies and I would lift weights, hoping the coeds were watching and basking in the feeling of burgeoning strength. Little did I know as a college student that there would come a time when, not only would I lack the hours to go to the gym to lift, but I wouldn't even have the space to set up the weights which had been collecting cobwebs for years. Even if I had the space, I would be paranoid about the free weights lying around with youngsters in the house.

One evening as I was playing with my youngsters, I playfully bench pressed Adam ten times. He loved it. Ellen, not wanting to be left out, began clamoring for her turn, so I obliged. That evening I went through the lifting routine my college partners and I used to do, using my children as the "live" free weights. I got an unbelievable workout, and the kids didn't want to stop. Even Daniel, who came through his surgery with all flags flying, loved to watch his siblings and Dad "play." As soon as he showed an interest in participating, he became a part of the fun. It started to become a nightly agreement with my children: they could play with Dad while he got a workout. We started calling it DADsercise.

As the days went on, I decided that it might be crazy, but I was going to make this a priority. I started experimenting with different ways to lift my children, keeping in mind the children's safety first and the targeted muscle groups second. I continued to run and walk when I could and actually ate what I thought was too much. The weight continued to fall off. Unbelievably, I could do no wrong when it came to dropping pounds. I had Old Mo' on my side — *mo*tions and actions specifically designed to strengthen my muscles and burn fat, *mo*mentum from the success I was experiencing, and *mo*tivation from my kids who acted as my personal trainers. Having my 3 year-old ask me to DADsercise was irresistible. How could I turn her down?

I decided that this idea was too good to keep to myself. I'm not a natural writer; I'm a computer programmer who can't spell. In fact, my high school English teacher will most likely fall off his chair when he sees that I wrote a book. Furthermore, throughout this book I never claim to be an expert on any diets, exercise regimens, or family counseling. I want this to be a testimonial on what worked and is working for me — how I came to discover through DADsercise an invigorating lifestyle, a newly-renovated body, and a special camaraderie with my children. I realize that as a parent my kids look to me as an example whether I want to be a role model or not. If they see me plopped on the couch every night, that's what they will want to do when given a choice. Discover what I did. Introduce exercise to your children at a young, impressionable age. The earlier children see their parents exercising and making wise health-conscious choices, the faster the children will develop a life-long love for exercise.

I want you to tell your wife that you can't afford the health club anymore, but that it has nothing to do with money but everything to do with family. I want you to tell your children to get ready to spend some time building on a project, a fun project called Dad! Get ready! Get set! Let's DADsercise!

The History of DADsercise

I still remember the exhilaration of getting on the floor with my dad, who, after coming in from hot days in the cornfields of central Nebraska, found time to roughhouse with his four children. He would tickle us to tears, wrestle with us, and delight us with his strength and ability to transform himself into a carnival ride. One particular ride would take one his kids from a sitting position on the floor to a vertigo-inducing four feet atop his foot. Only now, have I really thought about how much sheer strength he needed to lift each squirming child, balancing him or her perfectly. Not once did we fall. You can imagine the workout he got after each child begged for a turn; I don't remember his ever turning us down. Maybe he knew with his version of DADsercise over thirty years ago what I am now finally realizing: time spent with your children is priceless, a child's laugh is worth any cost, and a family that plays together will learn to play together for a lifetime. My siblings and I live in three different states but make it a priority to come back to our parents' home numerous times throughout the year to spend time together, to laugh, and to play. Did Dad have this in mind when he came home from the fields? Maybe. Maybe not. I just know how nostalgic I get when I think of the joyful romps we small children had with him.

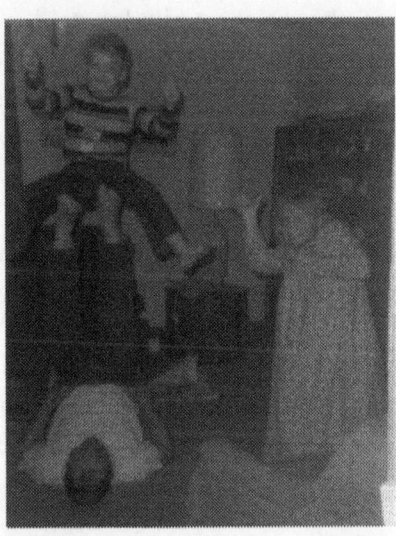

Time is a valuable commodity; where we invest our time will determine our rewards. But unlike money, time cannot be earned, it cannot be hoarded, it cannot be passed down from generation to generation, and in our lifetime it is not limitless. Our American work ethic often drives us to put off today's pleasures until tomorrow, but can we really afford to wait until we have enough to retire before we invest time with our children? I realize I have turned a little didactic here, but I have come to realize very poignantly that time spent away from my family can never be reinvested. Life slips away while we are making other plans to enjoy life. Malcolm Forbes' father once wrote "It isn't success if it costs you the companionship, chumminess, and love of your children." He came to realize that often the wealthiest men in the world "have sacrificed the finest thing in life, the affection of their family."

We all have a to-do list. What is at the top of your list? The year before Daniel's surgery and before my realization that I was neglecting my health, the majority of the items on my list would have been work related. Don't get me wrong. I still work many hours, but I have found that my list, now, includes much family time. Can I attribute this to my family's interest in DADsercise? I think back to my father, who, even though he didn't have access to a gym, wouldn't have sacrificed the time from his family anyway. I think back to my mother as she smiled watching her children climb on the mountain of her husband. She tells her adult children that she still cherishes those memories. DADsercise triggers a landmine of memories for me, too. Every time my wife watches or participates with us, her laughter rekindles those warm embers of nostalgia. Be assured, my wife and I have always stressed the need of spending time together as a family, but DADsercise has given my family a way to combine quality family time with a good old fashioned workout.

I have never had a personal trainer, but I can see how one would be very helpful. Trainers are patient, nurturing, persistent, and effective motivators. A good trainer knows that the human body is a sensitive machine, albeit mysterious at times, but he or she can find the right workout regimen for the client. Celebrity trainers, who can charge up to $300 an hour, put the names of J-Lo, Oprah, Madonna, and Tom Cruise in their appointment books. Some of the personal trainers, such as Bob Green, Oprah's trainer, and Gunter, trainer for many stars, have become as famous as their clients. They generate millions of dollars because they rub shoulders with the rich and famous. Their advice on diets and nutritional products makes many people much money; however, what may work for one person does not always work for another. There is no quick fix. Thousands of dieters have been frustrated by the blanket exercise routines and diet programs offered by the "experts" in the health industry.

At times I wonder how a personal trainer would match up to my kids. Their charge is room and board and lots of attention. Remember, to them this is fun. Resting is not fun. Taking turns is not fun. Stopping is not fun. When I get done with one kid on an exercise, the next one is ready for his or her turn. I'm not sure I could survive more kids.

Meet my personal trainers

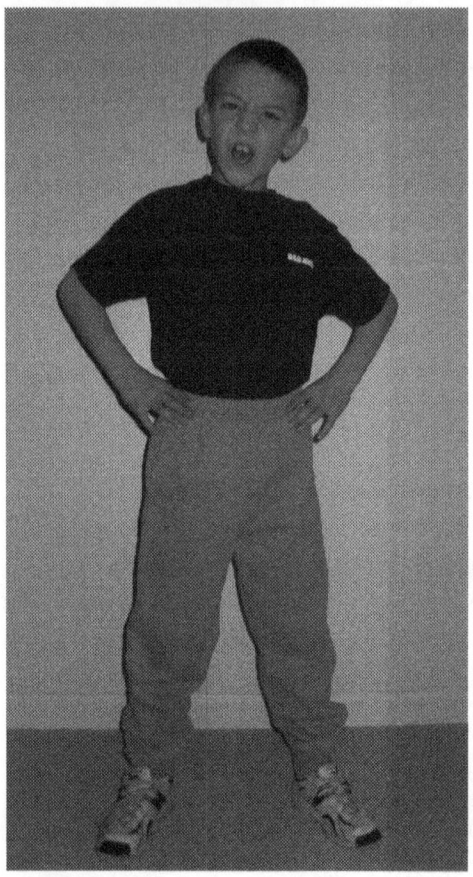

Name: Adam
Age: 8
Weight: 57 lbs.

Adam, my oldest child, is now starting to get a little too big for all the exercises, but he still has fun participating in DADsercise sessions. His training technique is to do the exercises with me, competing with me every sweat droplet of the way. Neither one of us likes losing, so we push each other pretty hard.

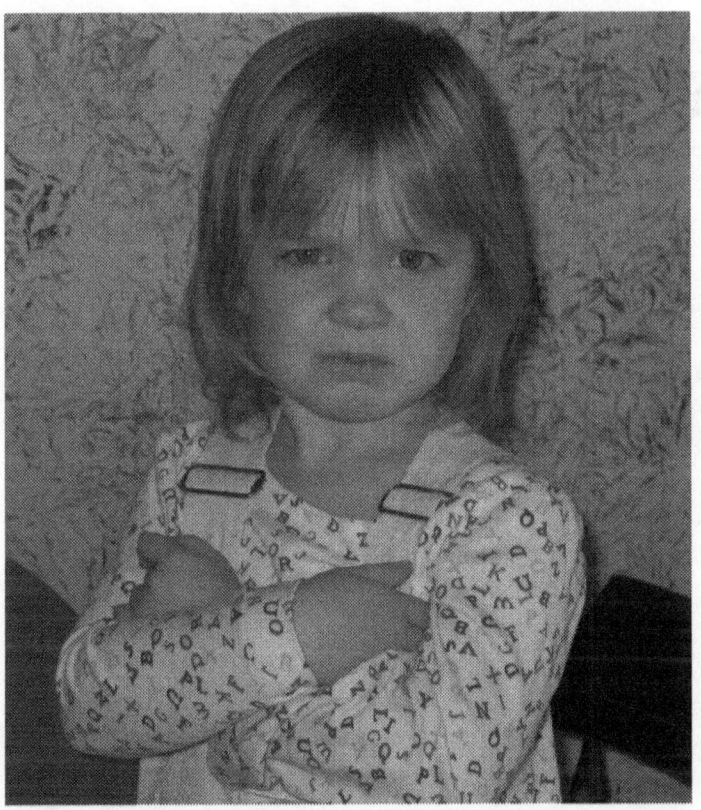

Name: Ellen
Age: 4
Weight: 34 lbs.

Ellen, my second child and only girl, is in the perfect age group
for DADsercising. Her training pattern consists of bombarding me
with energizing laughter and imperious demands. Her favorites
include "It's my turn!" and "Daddy, do the rocket with me!" My
favorite responses, after a few minutes with her are usually, "I just
did the rocket with you!" and "Can Daddy rest for just a second?"
Just guessing, but this is most likely not a technique used by
professional personal trainers, nonetheless, it is very effective.

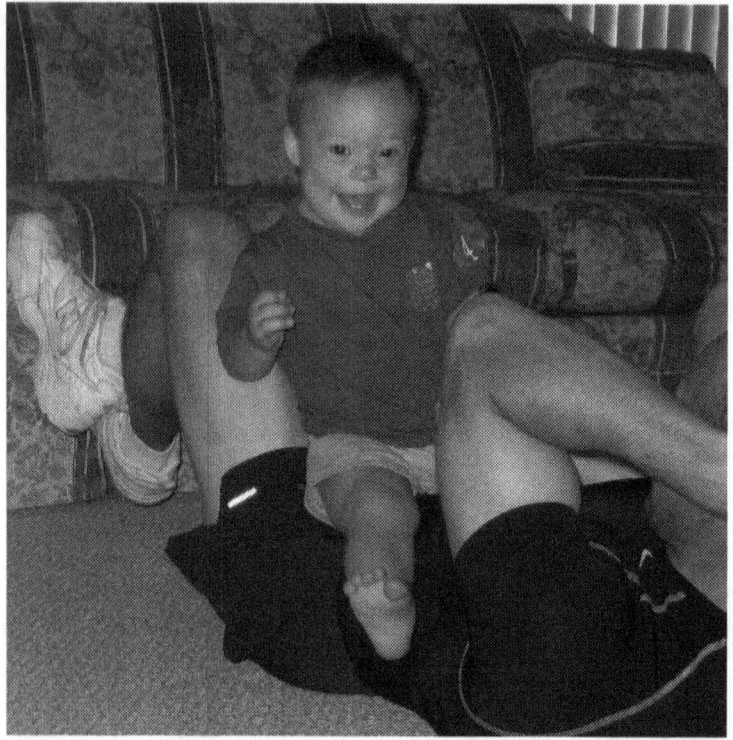

Name: Daniel
Age: 1
Weight: 24 lbs.

Even though Daniel is very young, he loves to DADsercise. Too young to talk, he has his ways of letting me know it's time to DADsercise. There have been times when I really didn't plan on DADsercising that night, but his body language lets me know that taking the night off is not in the cards. The smile on his face when I get down on the floor lights up the whole room.

One thing about children as personal trainers, everyone is different. I'm sure you will find out that your personal trainer may be very different from mine.

With demanding personal trainers and good exercise, you are bound to start dropping some of that weight. At this point in the description of any program, most authors would start discussing the details of their scientific, time-honored systems; however, I want to emphasize that DADsercise is not about detailing out a strict diet plan of what you should eat and what you shouldn't. All I ask is that if you want to take advantage of this exercise and lose some of that weight, you need to examine what and how much you are eating. Make a very conscious effort to eat right. Make a conscious effort to cut back on portions at the table. If you dish up everything you plan to eat onto your plate before you start eating and don't take seconds or thirds, you will be amazed as to how much less food your body can thrive on. This, however, does not mean that you won't be hungry at times between meals. Since your exercise level and metabolism rate will be going up with all this exercise, you will find that you need to eat a healthy snack. In opposition to current thought, I say you don't have to be hungry all the time to lose weight.

If you perceive DADsercise as a fad, your attempt to try it will be like a trip on the Titanic with ice ahead. DADsercise must be a life style change. Every day millions of people's days begin or end with a trudge off to some form of health club, tennis court, or jogging track. Once there, they work up a sweat and come home with the onset of soreness. If that were the scenario day in and day out, there would be no fitness issue in the United States. However, people don't stick to that regimen. Once they drag themselves home, their effort, sweat, and the majority of the benefit is undone by their lack of resolve at the table. Furthermore, the soreness is allowed to set in. Instead of exercising and stretching the sore muscles, which would greatly help with the onset of soreness, most people allow it to spread like a disease without taking any measures. Missing a few days becomes missing a few weeks and the vicious cycle will begin again once they go back to the workout. I can understand why some do not want to make this type of workout a lifestyle. I can assure you, your children will not let you skip this much. They will help you stay on track.

Is it safe?

You know yourself and your capabilities. Although you do not have to be in great shape to begin DADsercise, you need to be honest with yourself and your ability. You also know your kids. Do not do anything that either you or your kids do not feel comfortable doing. Determine sensibly how often and how long. Some basic guidelines should be followed:

- "No pain, No gain" is a myth (exercise should require effort, but not undue discomfort.)
- Watch your form and technique
- Warm up and cool down
- Use common sense, remember, this is supposed to be fun.
    - o Don't exercise too aggressively
    - o Don't go against doctor's orders. If you are new to exercise, consult your doctor to formulate a plan together.
    - o Don't endanger your child during any of the exercises (throwing them in the air)
    - o Perform DADsercise in an appropriate environment, preferably a soft padded floor. An exercise mat would be a great surface.

Getting Started

Like any well-organized and successful venture, a plan must be contrived. In your case, an exercise plan. I know how busy kids' schedules can get. You will have to put together a flexible schedule that will fit into your family's activities. Be prepared to change your plan often since activities change along with the seasons.

My plan starts with the basic goals that I try to accomplish each week. I try to have three cardiovascular workouts (running, walking, biking, swimming, aerobic wrestling exercises, etc.) and three weight (Kid) lifting workouts. How I accomplish this differs from week to week and season to season. I can't even begin to tell you how many different workouts I have had. Here are a few sample weeks that I have used throughout my DADsercise journey. (*Reproducible weekly charts can be found in the appendix of this book or at www.dadsercise.com*)

Before DADsercising: (EARLY SUMMER 2004)

I started my journey to lose weight upon returning home in late spring of 2004 from a twenty-year class reunion. I know that seems backwards. The typical pattern for most is to lose weight *before* a class reunion. Not me. I squeezed through the gymnasium door at 215 pounds, my heaviest ever. Embarrassed by my condition and determined to change my lifestyle after Daniel's surgery, I began by walking and running on the treadmill once I got home. I even ventured outside for a run on extended lunch breaks although running on pavement was difficult because I didn't have the treadmill pulling me along. Sometimes my family and I would go on a family fun walk. Adam and I would often take a football along to go out for passes down the sidewalk. This kept the walk from boring my son and added a little more exercise for both of us.

Before Dadsercising Workout Journal
(SAMPLE EARLY SUMMER WEEK)

DADsercise Daily Workout Journal						Set 1		Set 2		Set 3	
Day/Date	Exercise	Upper Body	Abs	Legs	Cardio	Child	Reps	Child	Reps	Child	Reps
Monday	Tread mill - 30 minutes				X						
Tues.	Off										
Wed.	Treadmill - 30 minutes				X						
Thurs.	Off										
Friday	Treadmill - 30 minutes				X						
Sat.	Family walk				X						
Sunday	Off										

Starting DADsercising (LATE SUMMER 2004)

After about three months of running and walking with a few
pushups mixed in from time to time, I was starting to feel a little
better about myself and had managed to lose a few pounds. I had,
however, hit somewhat of a wall, my weight loss coming to a
standstill. This is when I started DADsercising with my children,
exercising with them three times, sometimes even five times, a
week. When DADsercising two days in a row, I tried to target
different muscle groups. Targeting didn't always work, however,
since the kids had their favorite exercise and there was no denying
them. I maintained my running regimen three times a week,
sometimes outside, sometimes on the treadmill. Once I began to
lose weight again, I was able to increase my intensity and distance.
Soon, the routine began to feed upon itself. The more I exercised,
the more weight I lost. The more weight I lost, the easier it became
to exercise.

Starting DADsercise Workout Journal
(SAMPLE LATE SUMMER WEEK)

DADsercise Daily Workout Journal

Day/Date	Exercise	Upper Body	Abs	Legs	Cardio	Set 1 Child	Reps	Set 2 Child	Reps	Set 3 Child	Reps
Monday	Treadmill - 40 minutes				X						
	The Rocket	X		X		AS	10	ES	15		
	Pushups	X					40		30		20
	Single Wing	X				ES	10	ES	10		
	Windshield Wiper	X				ES	15				
	Press Time	X				AS	15	AS	15		
	Elevator	X				DS	10	DS	10		
Tuesday	The Rocket	X		X		ES	20	ES	15		
	Bow and Arrow	X					8		6		
	Pushups	X					30		20		
	Kid Situps		X			DS	20				
	Situps		X				20		20		
	Ultimate Crunch		X			ES	10				
	Squat			X		AS	20	AS	20		
	Front Lunge			X		DS	10	DS	10		
	Side Lunge			X		DS	10	DS	10		
Wed.	Treadmill 40 - minutes				X						
Thurs.	The Rocket	X		X		ES	20	ES	15		
	Single Wing	X				ES	20	ES	10		
	Press Time	X				AS	15	AS	15		
	Elevator	X				DS	10	DS	10		
	Windshield Wiper	X				ES	20	ES	15		
	Kid Stretch	X				ES	10	ES	10		
	Pushups	X					25		20		
Friday	Treadmill - 40 minutes				X						
	Squat			X		AS	20	AS	20		
	The Rocket	X		X		ES	20	ES	20		
	Kid Situps		X			DS	20				
	Situps		X				20		20		

DADsercise Daily Workout Journal

Day/Date	Exercise	Upper Body	Abs	Legs	Cardio	Set 1		Set 2		Set 3	
						Child	Reps	Child	Reps	Child	Reps
Fri (cont'd)	Ultimate Crunch		X			ES	10				
	Bounces		X			DS	2 minutes				
Sat.	off										
Sunday	Press Time	X				AS	15	AS	15		
	The Rocket	X		X		ES	20	ES	20		
	Kid Stretch	X				ES	10	ES	10		
	Elevator	X				DS	10	DS	10		
	Pushups	X					30		20		
	Squat			X		AS	20	AS	20		
	Single Wing	X				ES	20	ES	10		

Soccer and Wrestling Seasons (FALL 2004)

In the fall Adam participated in soccer and wrestling. Since I had to find a way to get my exercise and still get him to his activities, I decided to help out during his practices. In soccer the coach and I would scrimmage with the kids to help them with their technique. In wrestling practice I participated in the conditioning part of the practice, which replaced some of my requirements for a cardiovascular workout. I continued to DADsercise with the kids on other evenings and ran on the treadmill or did a living room cardiovascular workout with my son to complete my cardiovascular workouts. (I will explain the living room cardiovascular workout in more depth in a later chapter.) By the time wrestling was in full swing about the first of December, I had lost about 35 pounds. Adding DADsercise to my workout routine pushed me off the weight loss plateau that I had stalled out on. I had already exceeded my expectations and was starting to wonder how much I really could lose. To be honest, I was not really trying to lose weight anymore, I was just having fun.

Fall Season DADsercise Workout Journal (SAMPLE FALL WEEK)

DADsercise Daily Workout Journal

Day/Date	Exercise	Upper Body	Abs	Legs	Cardio	Set 1 Child	Reps	Set 2 Child	Reps	Set 3 Child	Reps
Monday	Wrestling Practice				X						
Tuesday	The Rocket	X		X		AS	6	ES	20	DS	15
	Praying Turtle	X				ES	8	ES	4		
	Single Wing	X				ES	10				
	Elevator	X				DS	15	DS	10		
	Hot Dog	X				ES	20	ES	15		
	Press Time	X				AS	20	AS	20		
	Situps		X				50		40		
	Ultime Crunches		X			ES	10	ES	10		
Wed.	Off										
Thurs.	Living Room Motion - 20 minutes				X	AS					
Friday	The Rocket	X		X		ES	20	DS	20	ES	10
	The Drink	X				ES	30	ES	20		
	Elevator	X				DS	15	DS	10		
	Hot Dog	X				AS	8	ES	20	ES	15
	Windshield Wiper	X				ES	20				
	Press Time	X				AS	20	AS	20		
Sat.	Run on Treadmill - 40 minutes				X						
	Side Lunge			X		DS	10				
	The Rocket	X		X		ES	20	DS	20		
	Squat			X		AS	30	AS	30		
	Front Lunge			X		DS	10				
	Kid Situps		X			DS	30				
	Ultimate Crunches		X			ES	10				
Sunday	The Rocket	X		X		ES	20	DS	20	ES	20
	Single Wing	X				AS	10	ES	10		
	The Drink	X				AS	30	ES	25		
	The Leaner	X				AS	15				

DADsercise Daily Workout Journal

Day/Date	Exercise	Upper Body	Abs	Legs	Cardio	Set 1 Child	Set 1 Reps	Set 2 Child	Set 2 Reps	Set 3 Child	Set 3 Reps
Sun (cont'd)	Windshield Wiper	X				ES	20				
	Situps		X				50		40		
	Crunches		X				20		15		
	Bounces		X	X		DS	2 minutes				

Cold Weather Workouts (WINTER 2004-05)

By the first of February, the wrestling season was over for my son. I had lost 45 pounds, within 10 pounds of my football-playing weight in high school, and I couldn't believe it. I would have never guessed that I even *had* 45 pounds to lose when I started. Although ecstatic I had lost the weight, I knew it wasn't time to stop. Adam, Ellen, and Daniel were still having fun with Dad, and I was not willing to sacrifice my time with them for anything. This was a lifestyle change that I would be reluctant to give up.

Cold weather seasons are the perfect time to DADsercise. Since the temperature is too cold to go outside, the kids have a lot of energy to expend. DADsercising is a perfect way to get rid of that extra energy. During these months we DADsercised five or six times a week, and I continued my cardiovascular workouts on the treadmill.

Winter Season DADsercise Workout Journal (SAMPLE WINTER WEEK)

DADsercise Daily Workout Journal

Day/Date	Exercise	Upper Body	Abs	Legs	Cardio	Set 1 Child	Reps	Set 2 Child	Reps	Set 3 Child	Reps
Monday	4 mile Treadmill run				X						
	The Eagle	X				ES	15	ES	10		
	Press Time	X				AS	20	AS	20		
	The Recliner	X				AS	15	AS	10		
	Hot Dog	X				ES	25	DS	20		
	Elevator	X				DS	10	DS	10		
	Shoulder Rolls	X				ES	20				
	Windshield Wiper	X				ES	20				
	Kid Situps		X			DS	30				
	Situps		X				40				
	Ultimate Crunches		X			ES	20				
Tuesday	Squat			X		AS	40				
	The Rocket	X		X		ES	20	DS	20		
	The Praying Turtle	X				ES	10	ES	10		
	Front Lunge			X		DS	10	DS	10		
	Side Lunge			X		DS	10	DS	10		
	Calf Raises			X		AS	20				
	Kid Stretch	X				ES	15	ES	10		
Wed.	4 mile Treadmill run										
Thurs.	The Rocket	X		X		ES	20	DS	20		
	Hot Dog	X				AS	5	ES	15		
	Elevator	X				DS	10	DS	10		
	Single Wing	X				ES	10	ES	10		
	Kid Situps		X			DS	30				
	Crunches		X				20				
	Rock, Paper, Scissors		X				30				
	Popcorn			X	X	ES	20	ES	20		
	Tag Team Stairs			X	X	AS	10	AS	10	AS	10
	Helicopter				X	AS	10	AS	10		
Friday	OFF										

15

DADsercise Daily Workout Journal

Day/Date	Exercise	Upper Body	Abs	Legs	Cardio	Set 1 Child	Reps	Set 2 Child	Reps	Set 3 Child	Reps
Sat.	4 mile Treadmill run				X						
Sunday	The Rocket	X		X		ES	20	DS	20		
	Squat			X		AS	40	AS	20		
	Front Leg Lifts			X		ES	20	ES	20		
	Reverse Leg Lifts			X		AS	10	AS	10		
	The Drink	X				ES	30	ES	30		
	Hot Dog	X				ES	25	ES	20		
	Elevator	X				DS	10	DS	10		
	Kid Pull over	X				ES	10	ES	10		

Warmer Weather Workouts (Late Spring/ Early Summer 2005)

Someone once said that the only difference between a jogger and a runner is an entry form. In the spring I set a goal to run a 10K road race; in the summer I filled out the entry form. This upcoming fall event has not only motivated me to intensify my cardiovascular workouts, but it has given my "new" persona a chance to slam the door on my old perceptions of myself.

Spring and summer evenings seem to be busier than any other evenings for my family: baseball practice, bike riding, or the kids playing in the yard. To intensify my cardiovascular workout, I would get up early in the morning before work to run, which helped me beat the heat of the day. Since the kids were not always as available during the spring and summer, I either shortened my workouts with them or sometimes only worked out with them a few times a week. To make up for this, I did exercises that I could do without them (pushups, sit ups, crunches, etc.) in the evening after they went to bed.

Warm Weather Season DADsercise Workout Journal (SAMPLE WARM WEATHER WEEK)

DADsercise Daily Workout Journal

Day/Date	Exercise	Upper Body	Abs	Legs	Cardio	Set 1 Child	Reps	Set 2 Child	Reps	Set 3 Child	Reps
Monday	Morning Hill Run - 5 miles				X						
	Situps		X				50		40		
	Rock, Paper, Scissors		X				20		20		
	Crunches		X				20		20		
	The Rocket	X				ES	20	DS	20		
	Pushups	X					50		50		
	Hot Dog	X				DS	30	DS	30		
	Elevator	X				DS	10				
Tuesday	Morning 4 mile easy run				X						
	Evening Swimming with children				X						
Wed.	Morning 6 mile run				X						
	Situps		X				50		40		
	Rock, Paper, Scissors		X				20		20		
	Crunches		X				20		20		
	Front Lunge			X		DS	10	DS	10		
	Side Lunge			X		DS	10	DS	10		
	Front Leg Lift			X		DS	10	DS	10		
Thurs.	Morning 4 mile easy run				X						
	Evening Family Bike Ride				X						
Friday	Hot Dog	X				ES	20	DS	30		
	Elevator	X				DS	10	DS	10		
	Eagle	X				AS	20	ES	20		
	The Drink	X				ES	20	ES	20		
	The Leaner	X				AS	20	ES	20		
	The Recliner	X				AS	20				
	Kid Situps		X			DS	30				
	Crunches		X				20		20		
	Perch		X			ES	20				
	Loader		X			DS	20				

17

DADsercise Daily Workout Journal										
		Upper Body	Abs	Legs	Cardio	Set 1		Set 2		Set 3
Day/Date	Exercise					Child	Reps	Child	Reps	Child	Reps
Sat.	Morning 6 mile run				X						
Sunday	Hot Dog	X				ES	20	DS	20		
	Elevator	X				DS	10	DS	10		
	The Drink	X				ES	30	ES	20		
	Press Time	X				AS	20	AS	20		
	Windshield Wiper		X			ES	30				
	Spider		X			ES	20				
	Squat			X		AS	40	As	30		
	Front Leg Lifts			X		ES	20	DS	20		
	Calf Raises			X		AS	20				
	Reverse Leg Lifts			X		AS	10	ES	10		

Admittedly, it is not always easy to come up with a plan during this time frame to get your exercise. Sometimes you have to be creative. At the beginning of the week, I would check the family activities, envisioning how I could fit my exercise into them. Sometimes my plan would work, sometimes it wouldn't. As I mentioned earlier, if activities prevent you from exercising with your kids, you can always fall back on pushups and sit ups. If done passionately, they will be enough to keep you going, your body tuned for when your kids are next available.

SETTING GOALS

While planning what will work for you and your family, you need to talk to your kids about what you are trying to do. Explain to them how important their role will be in shaping a new dad. Kids love to help out, especially when it involves having fun.

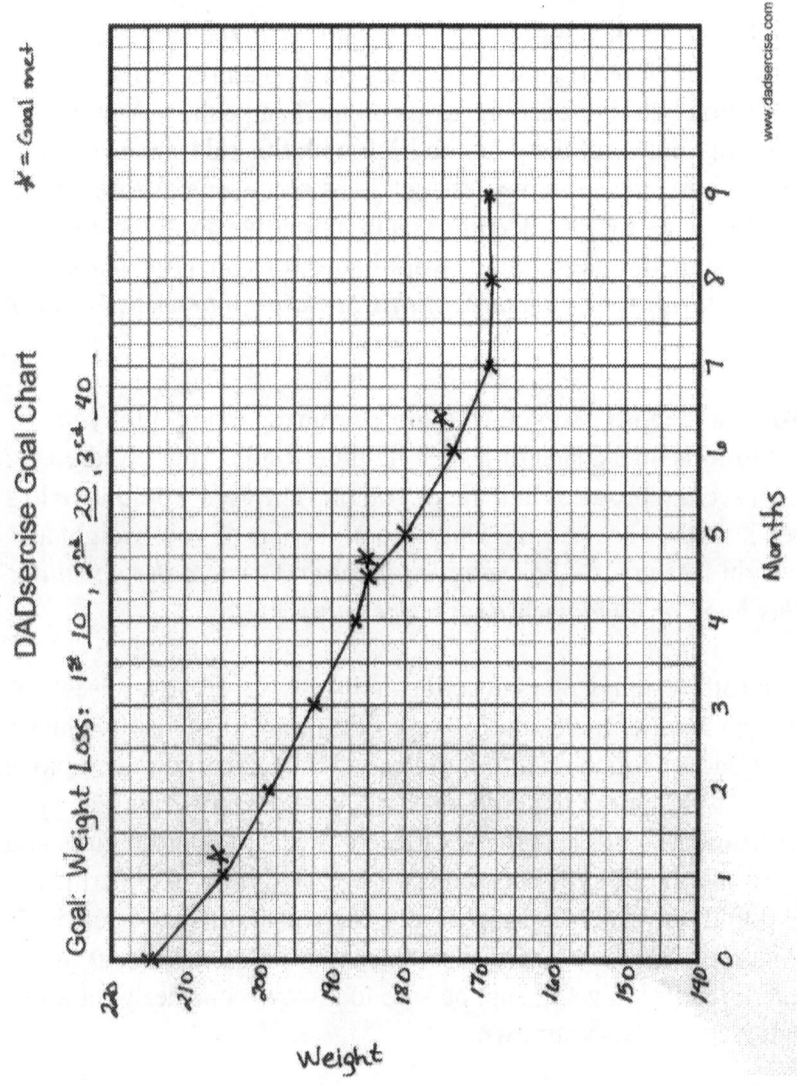

DADsercise Goal Chart

✗ = Goal met

Goal: Weight Loss: 1ˢᵗ _10_ , 2ⁿᵈ _20_ , 3ʳᵈ _40_

www.dadsercise.com

Weight

Months

19

Your children's involvement in the goal setting can be an important lesson in life. As adults out in the "real world," we understand the importance of goal setting, either intrinsically or extrinsically. I suggest that you create personal short-term and long-term goals, but let your children take ownership in many of the goals as well. After I reached a certain number of pushups with my children on my back, we all went out for ice cream. With ice cream on the line, my children counted out every pushup and screamed with joy when I straightened my arms on the last pushup. A word of warning: don't set the goal too high with the kids since you want to reach it. Once you meet the goal, set a new one. Although ice cream works for us since this is a treat that we don't have very often, something else might work better for you. (***For blank goal charts turn to the appendix of this book or go to www.dadsercise. com***)

To give the kids and you a tangible progress report, plot your repetitions on a chart for a specific time frame. Your children can then see the progress and cheer you on. The kids would love to see how they are helping Dad on a plot chart of your weight and weight loss goals. (***For sample plot charts turn to the appendix of this book or go to www.dadsersice.com***)

The following chapters describe and show several exercises that my personal trainers and I have used to transform Perry Schnacker, complacent couch potato, into Perry Schnacker, motivated pioneer. Some we do more than others, some we do every time. Each child is different—different sizes, different levels of coordination, and most of all, different personalities. You will have to experiment and find out which exercises work for you and which ones don't. Please use all these exercise as starting points. Make your own exercises if you want. Just be sure to always consider your kids' safety as well as your own.

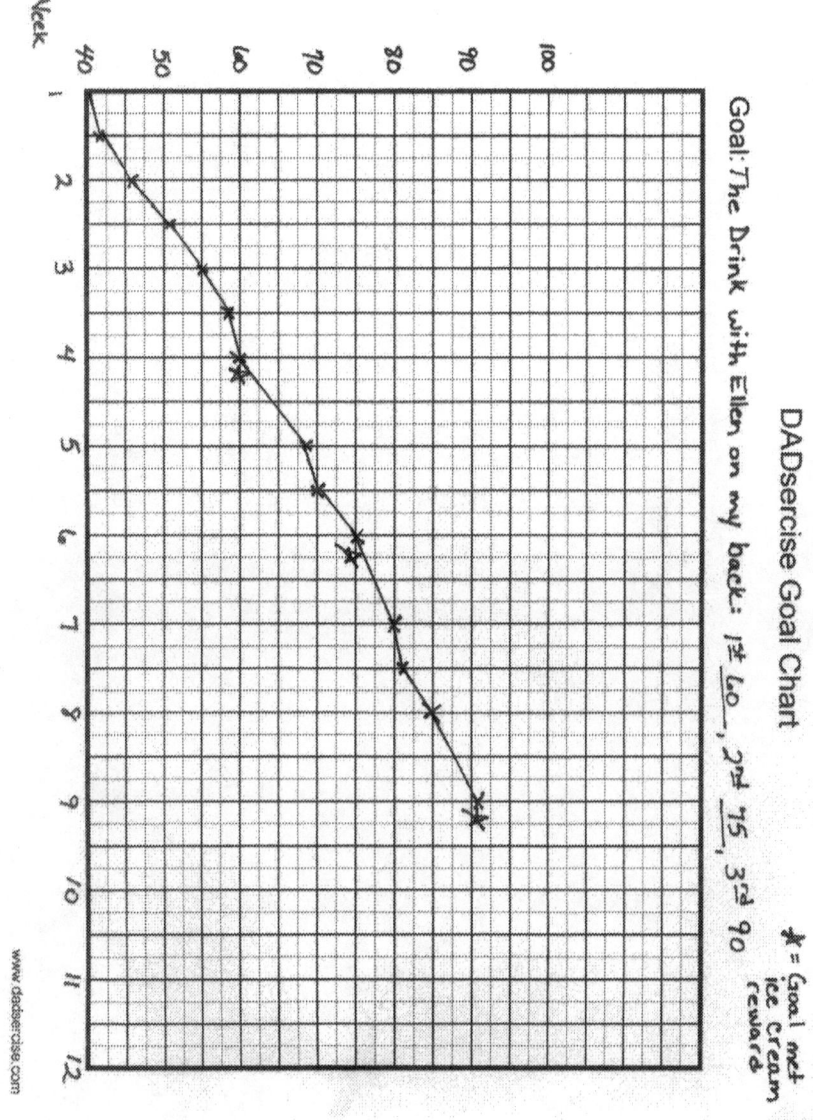

DADsercise Goal Chart

Goal: The Drink with Ellen on my back: 1ˢᵗ 60 , 2ⁿᵈ 75 , 3ʳᵈ 90

✱ = Goal met
    ice cream
    reward

www.dadsercise.com

21

Ok, it's time. Look at your schedule, talk to your kids, put together a plan, and get started.

Stretching

While DADsercise can seem like playing, it is also strenuous exercise. All good exercise programs use stretching to prevent injury and prepare the body for work. I have listed a few of the stretches that I do before exercising. Please do not skip this step. In fact, have your children join in to make it even more fun.

Ankle Pull

Thighs

- Lay on the floor face down.
- Reach back and grab your ankle and gently pull it towards your buttocks until you feel pressure. Make sure the heel is directly in line with the buttocks since knees can suffer from wrong angles.
- Hold for the count of ten and then repeat with the other leg.
- If you have trouble reaching your ankle, wrap a towel around your ankle and pull on the towel.
- This stretch can also be done standing up. Be sure to support yourself with your free hand when performing this stretch.

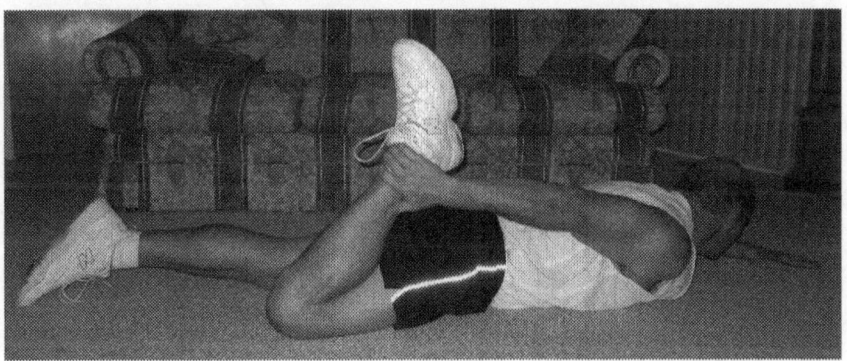

Touch Toes

Hamstrings and Lower Back

- Sit on the floor with your legs basically straight. (There is no need to lock out the knees)
- Reach out for your toes until you feel pressure in the hamstrings.
- Hold for a count of ten and repeat.

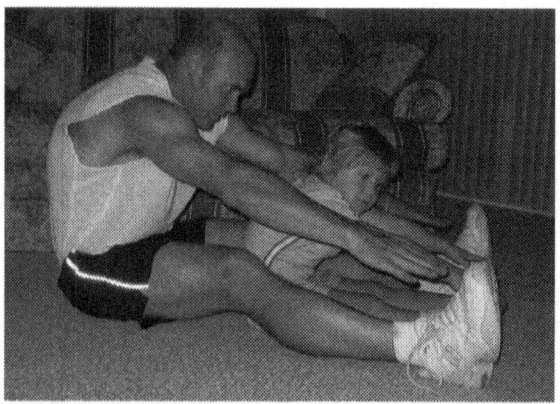

Crossover

Upper Hamstrings and Hips

- Sit on the floor and cross one leg over the other with your knee in the air.
- Place your elbow from the opposite arm on your knee.
- Twist your body until you feel pressure and hold for a count of ten and then repeat with the other side.

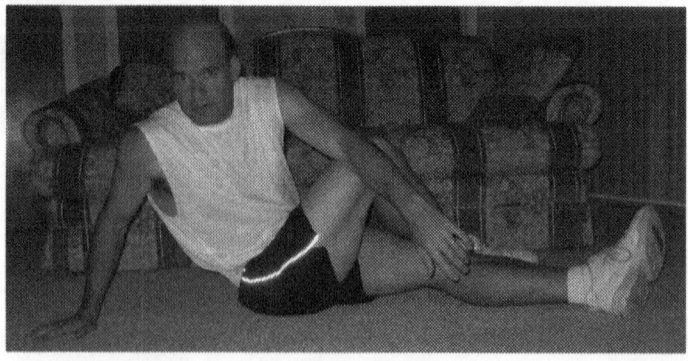

Wall Push

Calves

- Place your hands on a wall and extend one leg behind you.
- Lower yourself until you feel pressure on your calf muscle.
- Hold for the count of ten and then repeat with the other leg.
- Repeat while bending back leg, keeping heel down

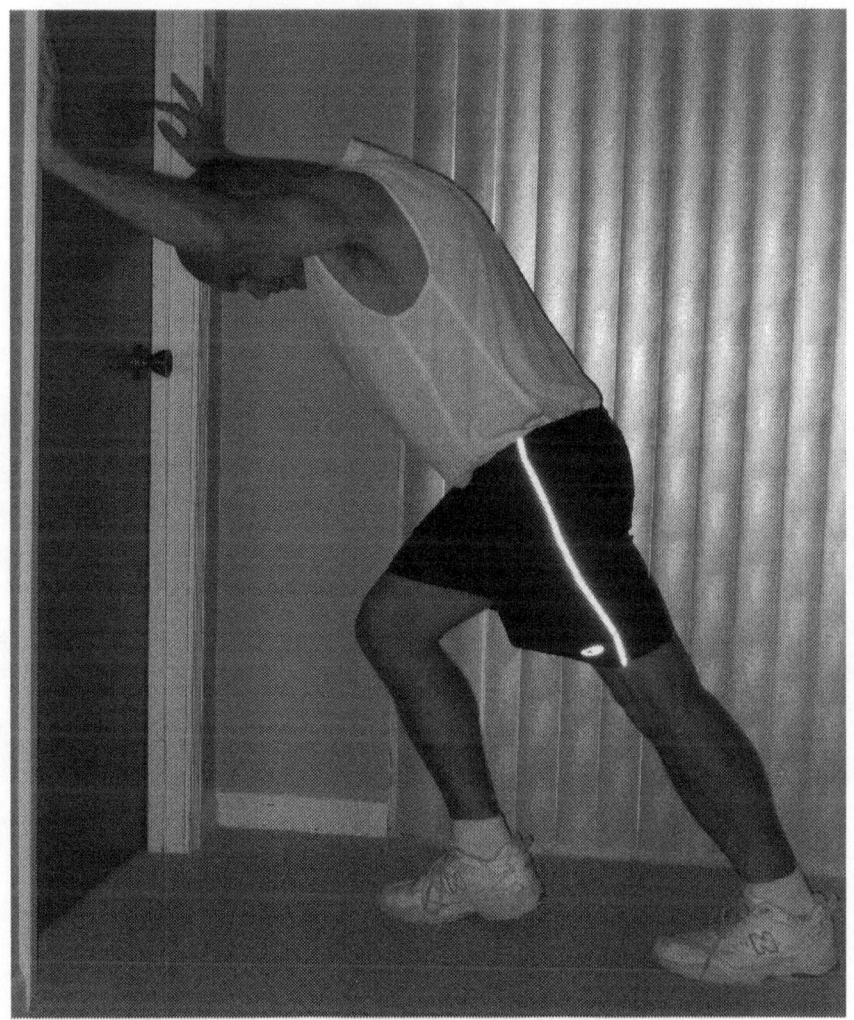

Chest Stretch

Chest and Shoulder

- Grab a doorway frame with your arm extended to your side.
- Gently twist your body until you feel pressure across your chest.
- Hold for the count of ten and repeat on the other side.

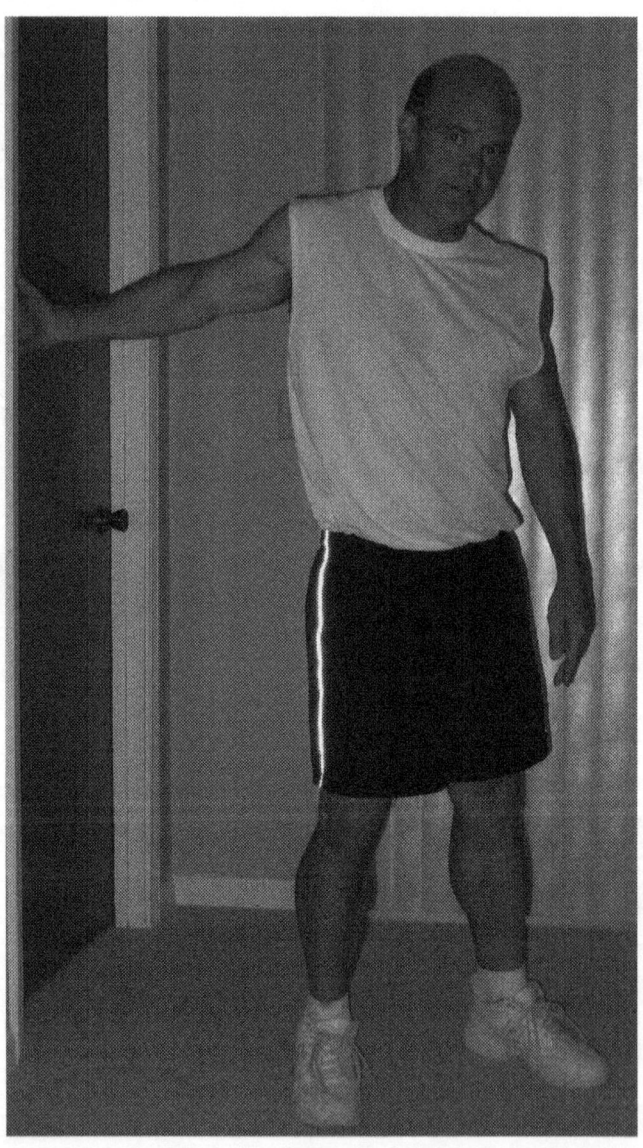

Down the Back

Arms and Side

- Lift one arm behind your head and reach your hand down your back.
- Grab your elbow with your other hand and gently apply pressure, pushing your hand down your back.
- Hold for the count of ten and repeat on the other side.

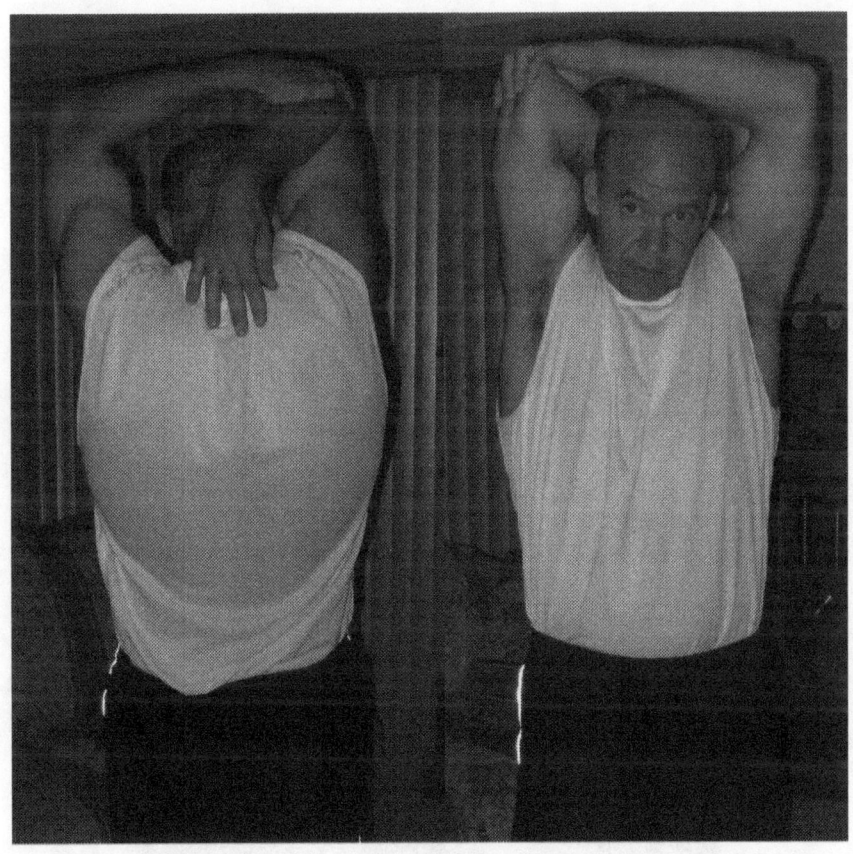

Arm Pull

Arms, Shoulders, and Side

- Lift an arm behind your head with the hand coming over your other shoulder.
- Grab your elbow with the other hand and pull gently until you feel pressure.
- Hold for a count of ten and then repeat with the other arm.

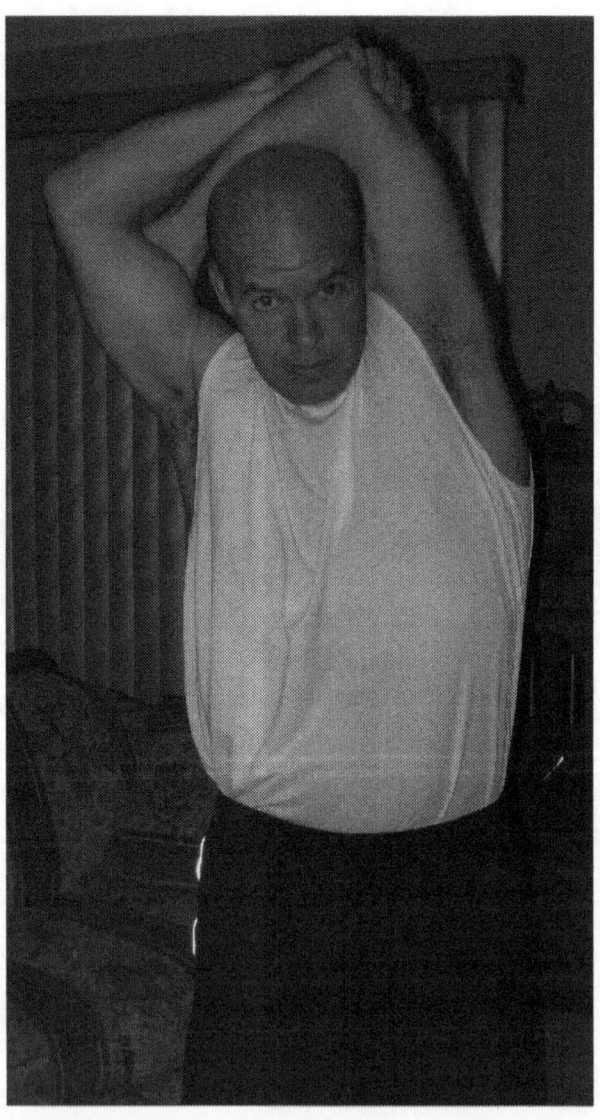

Shoulder Stretch

Shoulders

- Extend your arm in across your chest.
- Grab your elbow with the other hand and gently pull your arm toward your chest.
- Pull until you feel pressure in your shoulder and hold.
- Repeat with the other arm.

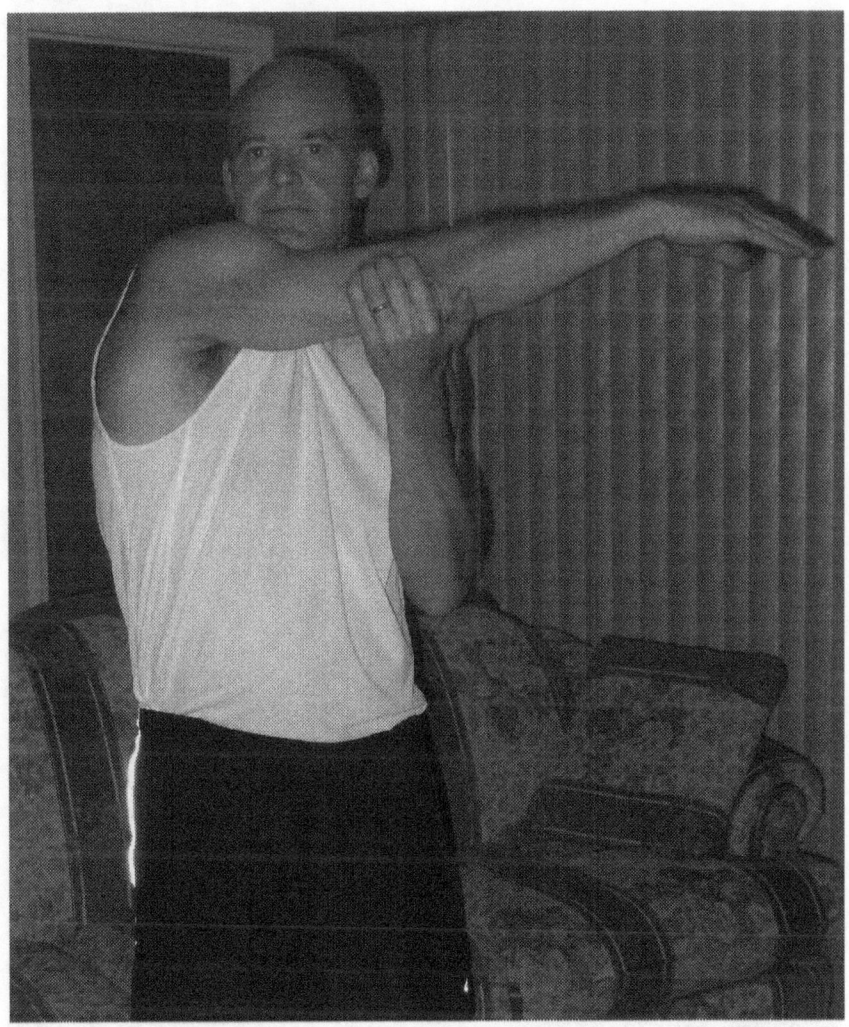

Neck Stretch

Neck

- Place one arm behind your back.
- Gently pull you head to the side with your other hand.
- Tilt your head until you feel a gentle stretch.
- Hold for a count of five.
- Repeat for the other side.

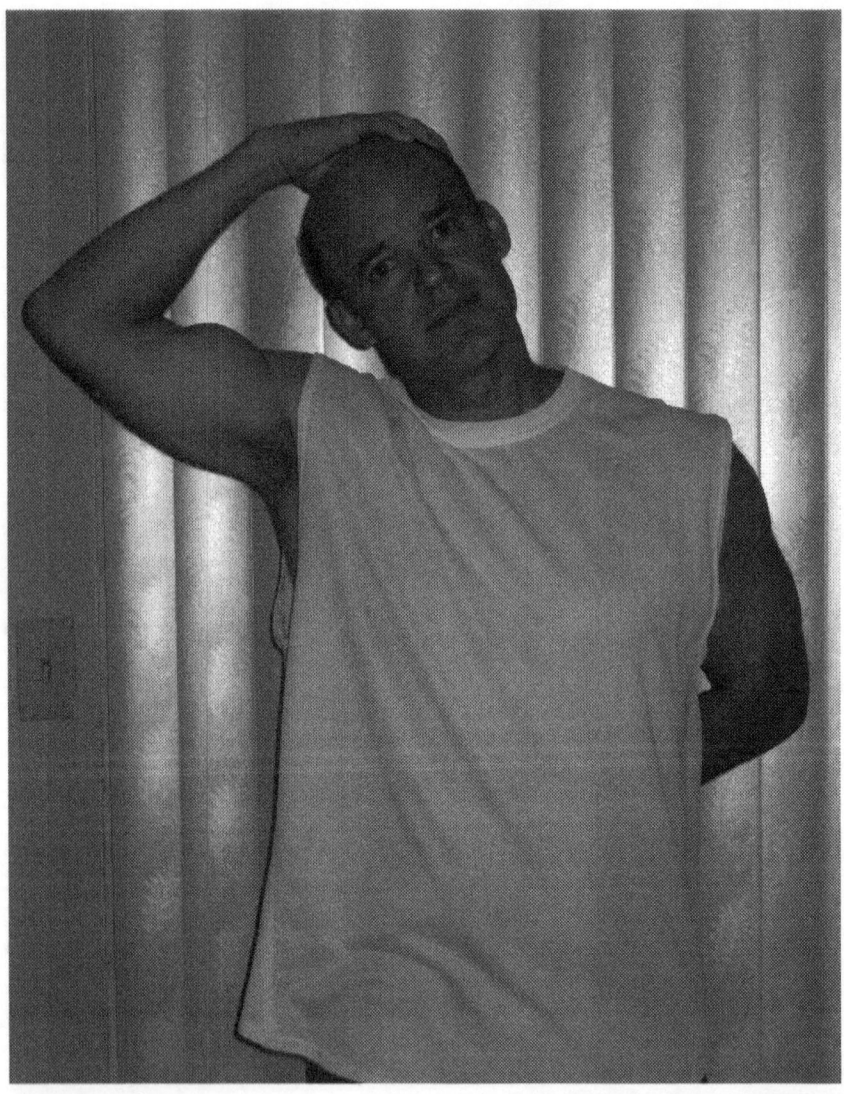

Upper Body Exercises

Basic Pushup

Arms and Chest

- Lie on the floor with your hands placed just outside your shoulders.
- Raise yourself up, keeping your back straight with your toes on the ground.
- Lower your chest back to the ground, again, keeping your back straight.
- Continue until your repetition goal is met.

If you find it difficult to do very many pushups in the beginning, try doing this pushup from your knees instead of your toes. This makes the pushup a little easier.

I have had my kids ride on my back from time to time but have decided that it puts too much pressure on my back. There are other variations of the pushup defined later in which your kids can actively participate by riding. Nevertheless, encourage your kids to join you by doing pushups themselves.

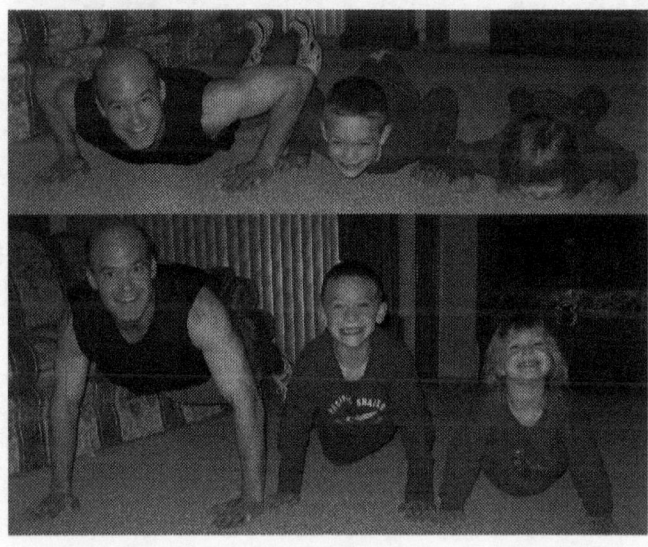

The Bow and Arrow

Arms and Chest

- Start in the up position.
- Join your thumbs and pointer fingers together so that the fingers create a triangle.
- Lower yourself down, bringing your nose down into the finger triangle.
- Be sure to keep your back straight.
- Raise yourself back up and continue until your repetition goal is met.

I find this exercise more strenuous than the basic pushup. Again, I would not recommend children on the back during this exercise.

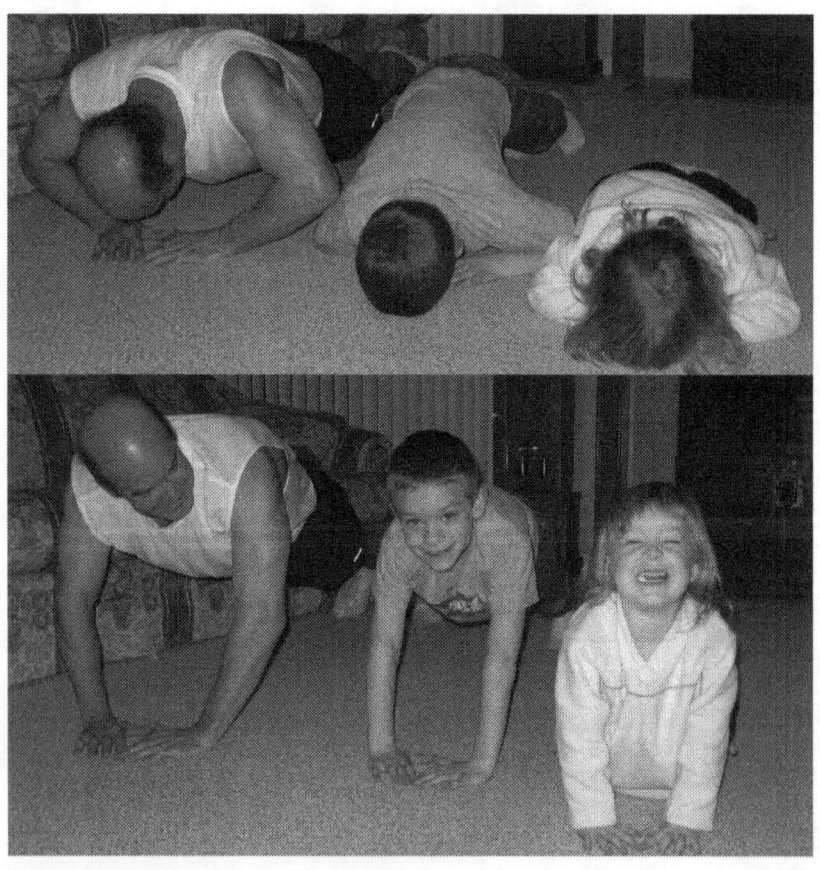

The Praying Turtle

Arms and Chest

- Start in the up position with the derriere up in the air.
- Join the thumbs and pointer fingers together so that the fingers create a triangle.
- (optional) Have your child climb on and hang on. If your child does not feel safe, have them stand on the back of your legs instead of lying on your back.
- Lower yourself down, bringing the nose down into the finger triangle.
- Be sure to keep your back straight.
- Raise yourself back up and continue until your repetition goal is met.

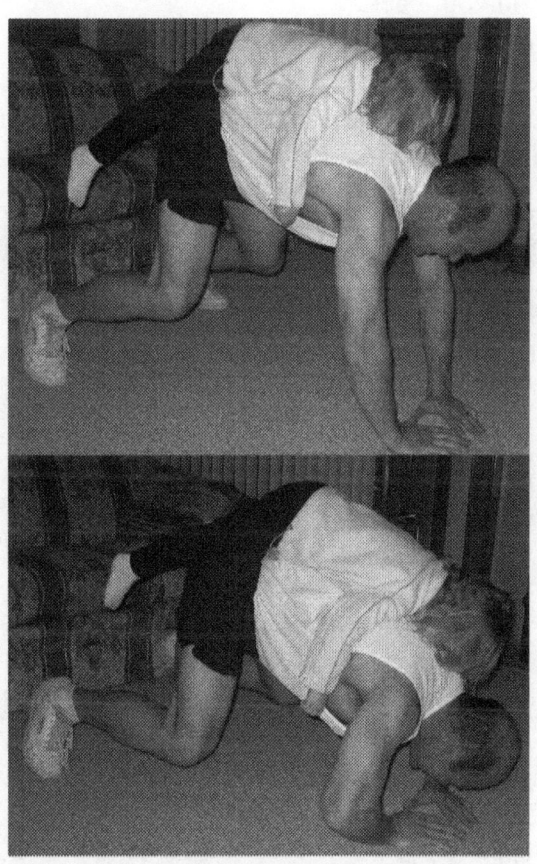

The Eagle

Arms and Chest

- Do not perform this exercise if you have any shoulder problems. Adding the weight of your child might not be a good idea if you have any concern about your shoulder strength.
- Place three sturdy chairs, or two chairs and a couch, in a triangle. Be sure the chairs are sturdy. You don't want to end up in a pile of chair and flesh.
- Place each hand on a chair and then the feet, or knees, on the third.
- (Optional) Have one of your kids get on your back and hang on. If you decide to have a child ride on your back, you will want to place your knees on the couch or chair. This puts less pressure on your back.
- Lower yourself down between the chairs.
- Push yourself back up.
- When your repetition goal is met, simply walk your feet off the couch to the ground and have your child get off.

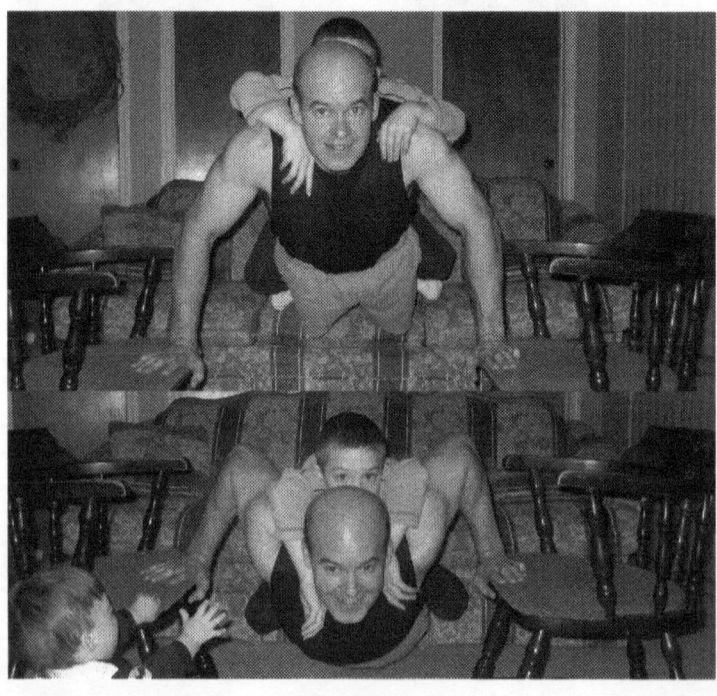

The Drink

Arms and Chest

- Place your knees on a couch.
- (optional) Have your child climb on your back and hang on.
- Lower yourself down, bringing the nose almost to the floor.
- Raise yourself back up until the arms are straight again.
- When your repetition goal is met, bring your knees to the floor and have your child crawl off.

This is a good exercise for goal setting since the children can actively participate.

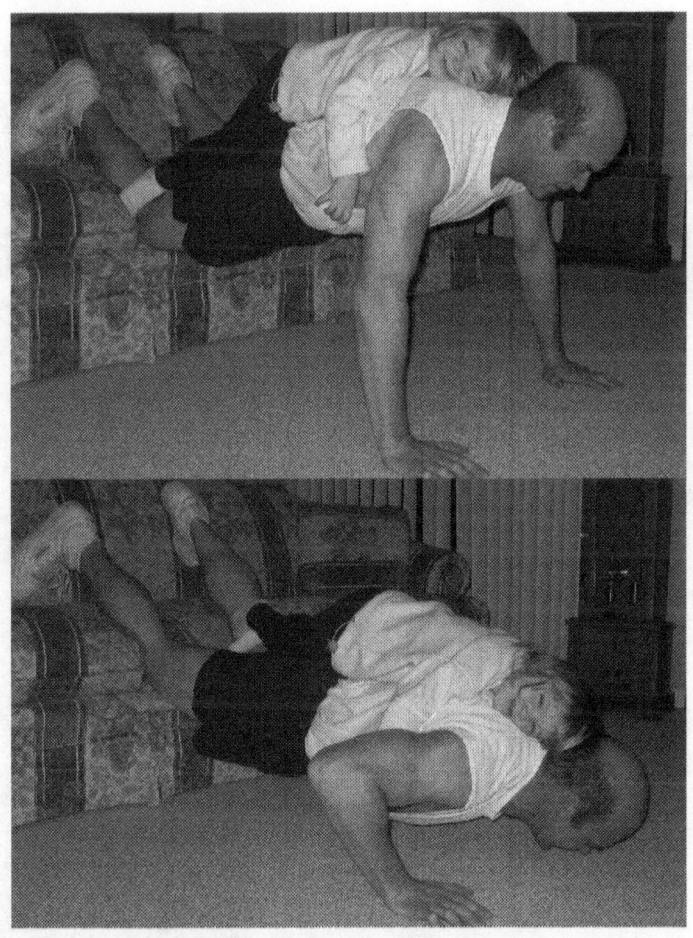

The Single Wing

Arms and Chest

- Place one arm on a chair and the other on the floor. Be sure to use a sturdy chair.
- (optional) Have your child climb on your back and hang on.
- Raise yourself up
- Lower yourself down so that your arm on the floor creates a 90 degree angle.
- Once you perform the desired number or repetitions on one side, switch to the other.
- My son Adam came up with this one.

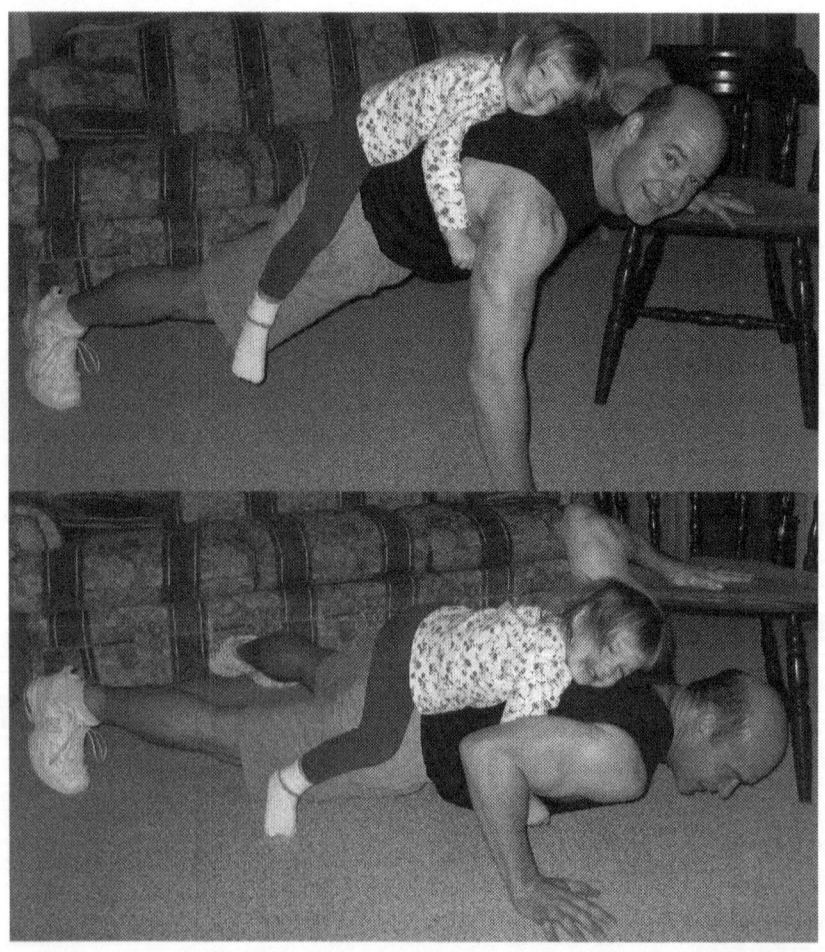

The Recliner

Arms

- With your back to a chair, place both hands on a chair. Be sure that you use a sturdy chair.
- (optional) Have your child sit on your lap.
- Lower yourself as low as you can comfortably go.
- Raise yourself back up.
- Continue until your repetition goal is met.

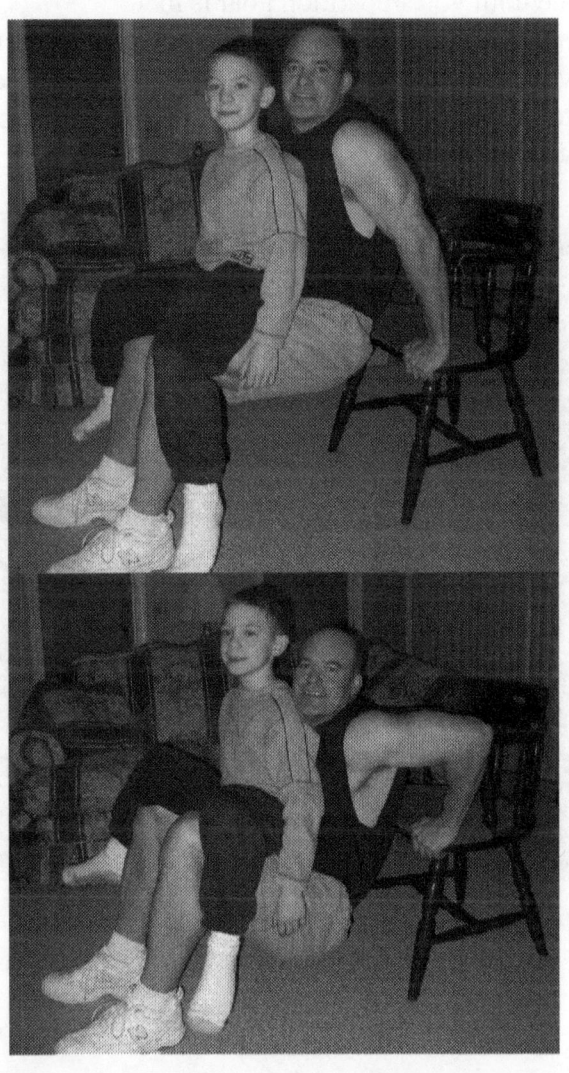

The Leaner

Arms and Chest

- (optional) Have your child climb on your back.
- Place your hands on each side of a doorway.
- Move your feet back until you are at a comfortable angle.
- Come forward between the door frames, making sure to stretch the chest muscles.
- Push yourself back to the starting position.
- Continue until your repetition goal is met.
- You need to find a doorway that you are able to reach both sides without extending your arms too wide. The doorway also needs to not be too narrow so that you are comfortable coming in between the two frames.

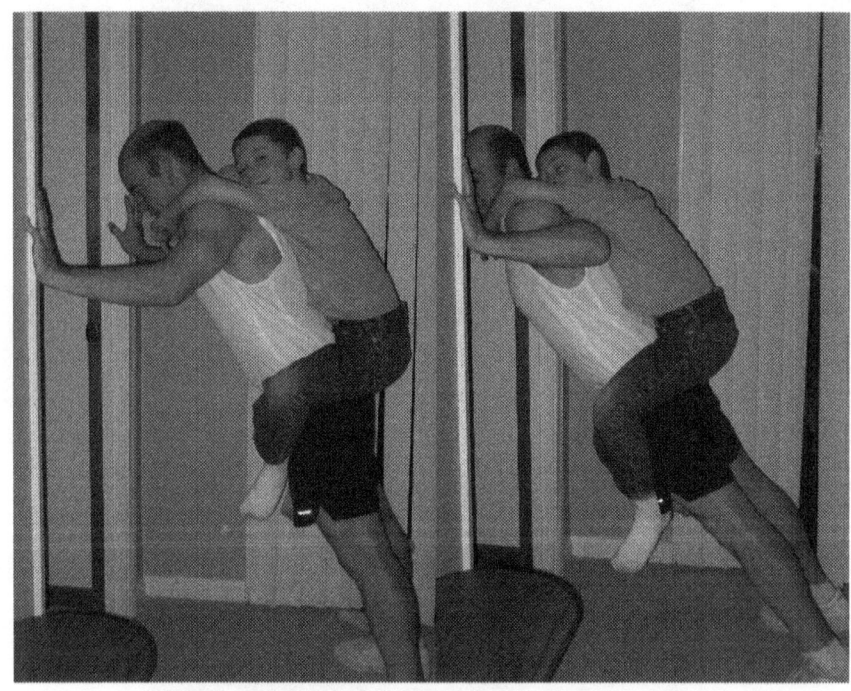

Press Time

Arms and Chest

- Lie with your back on the floor.
- Have your child stand beside you.
- Place one hand between his or her shoulder blades and the other on his or her derriere.
- Have the child lean back and relax. It is much easier to balance your children if they lay their head back in a relaxed position.
- Raise your child to the top position.
- Lower your child back to your chest.
- Perform as many repetitions as you can. You might find that you are working one arm a little more than the other.
- Have your child come around to the other side to even the discrepancy and go again.
- I simply stand my child up when done by lowering my hand under the derriere and raising the one under the back.

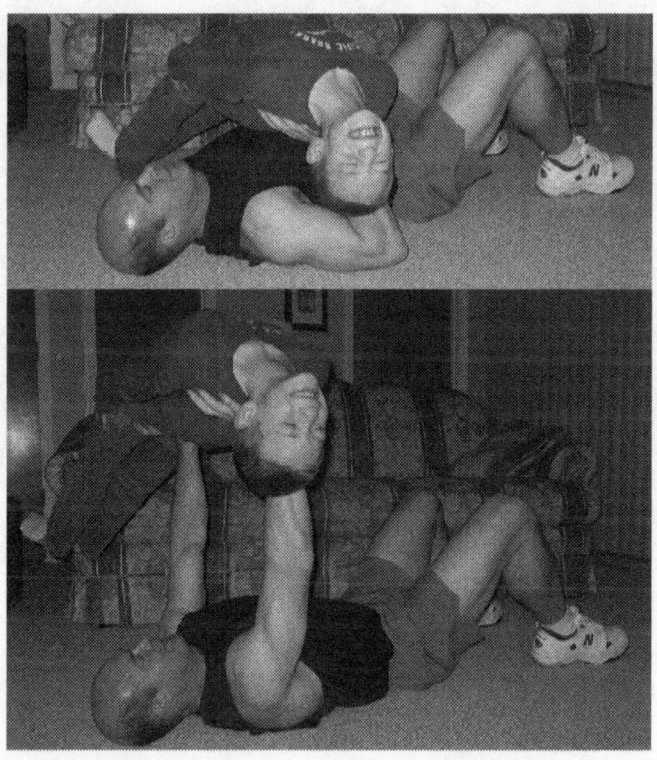

Elevator

Arms

- Pick up your child and place one hand under the arm and the other under the derriere.
- Be sure to hang on to your child well with the hand under the arm.
- Lower your child, bringing your arm to a straight position.
- Raise your child, concentrating on working the bicep muscle.
- Switch sides to work both biceps better.
- Continue until the desired repetitions are done.
- Doing this exercise in front of a mirror is fun for the child.

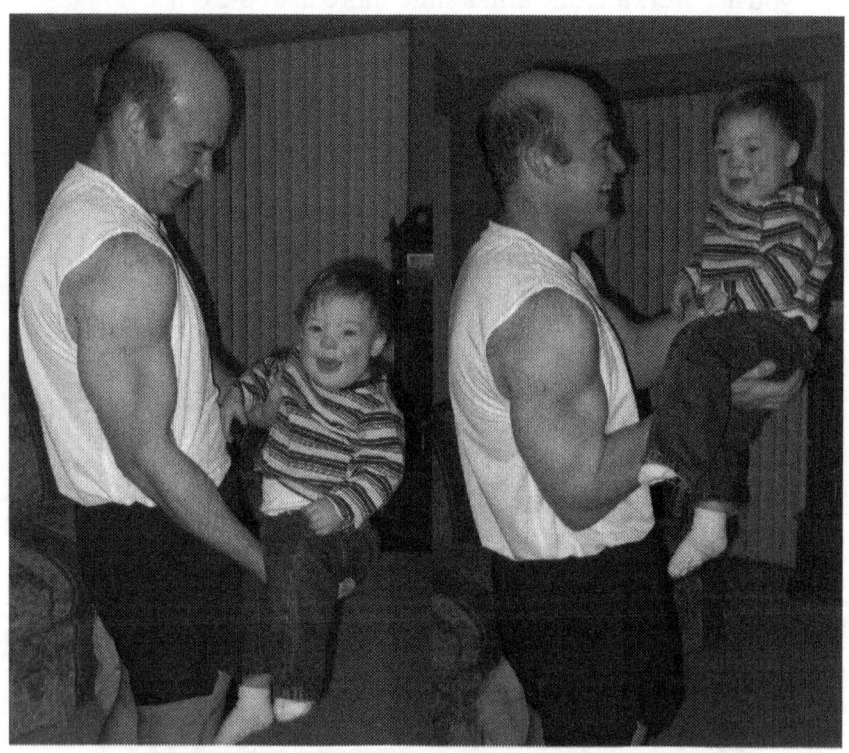

Hot Dog

Arms

- Sit on a couch or a chair.
- Lay a towel on the floor in front of you.
- Have your child lie on the towel.
- Bring both ends of the towel together and then roll them up.
- Roll them so that the fingers will be rolled up into the towel when lifting.
- Raise your child, trying to concentrate on using the biceps to do the lifting.
- Lower and go again until your repetition goals are done.
- My kids fight for turns on this exercise.

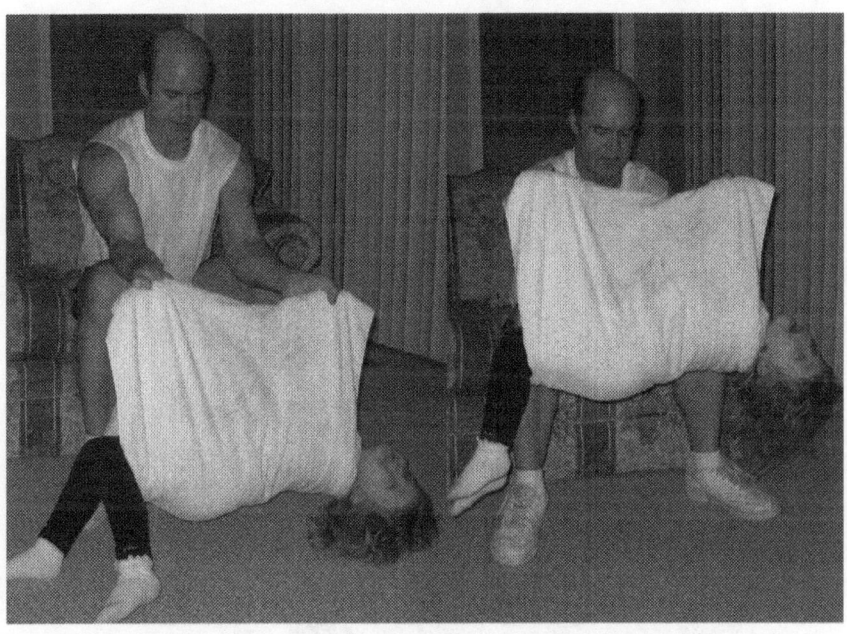

The Windshield Wiper

Arms and Chest

- Lie with your back on the floor.
- Have your child come from the side and pick him or her up from under the legs.
- When I do this with my older son, I have him hold his feet. This seems to help both of us keep our balance.
- Keep your lower back on the floor.
- Keeping your arms straight, bring the child over your head so his or her feet almost touch the floor.
- Return to the starting position and continue until the repetition goal is met.

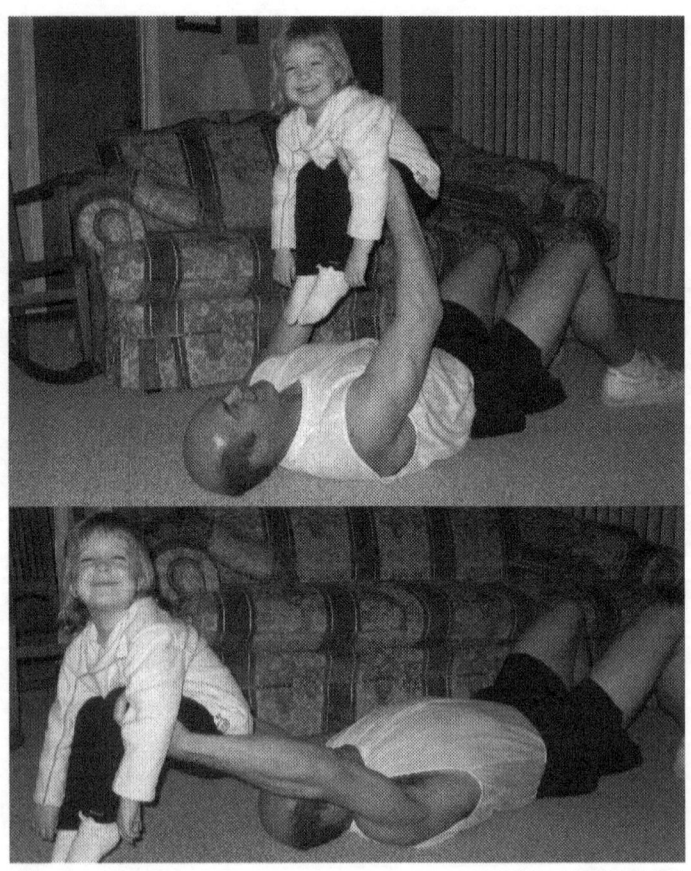

Half Rocket

Arms and Shoulders

- Pick up your child and hold him or her under the arms.
- Raise your child as high as you can.
- Return your child to the starting position and continue until the repetition goal is achieved.
- ***Don't throw your child up in the air**. You can give him or her the sensation of being thrown by lifting up quickly and then coming down quickly. Be sure to watch your child's reaction to be sure that he or she enjoys this fast action.

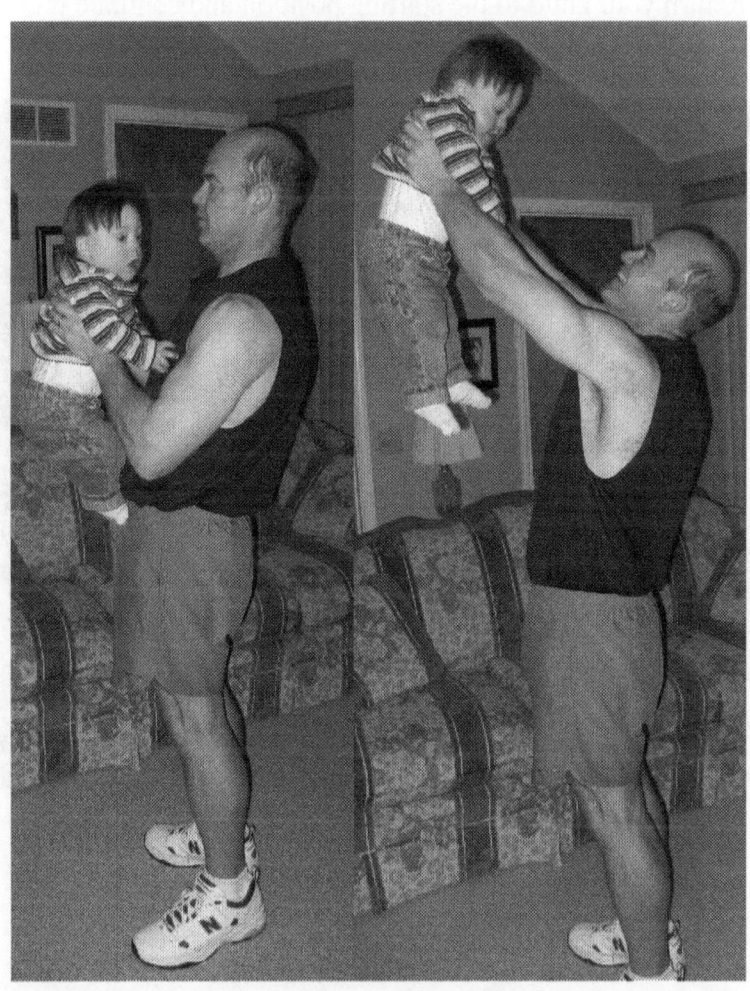

Kid Pull over

Arms

- Lie with your back to the floor.
- Have your child stand beside you and then have him or her lean back while you place one hand in the middle of the upper back and the other on the derriere.
- Lift him or her up over yourself until your arms are straight.
- Keep your lower back on the floor.
- Bending your arms, bring your child down to the top of your head.
- Return your child to the starting position and continue until the repetition goal is met.

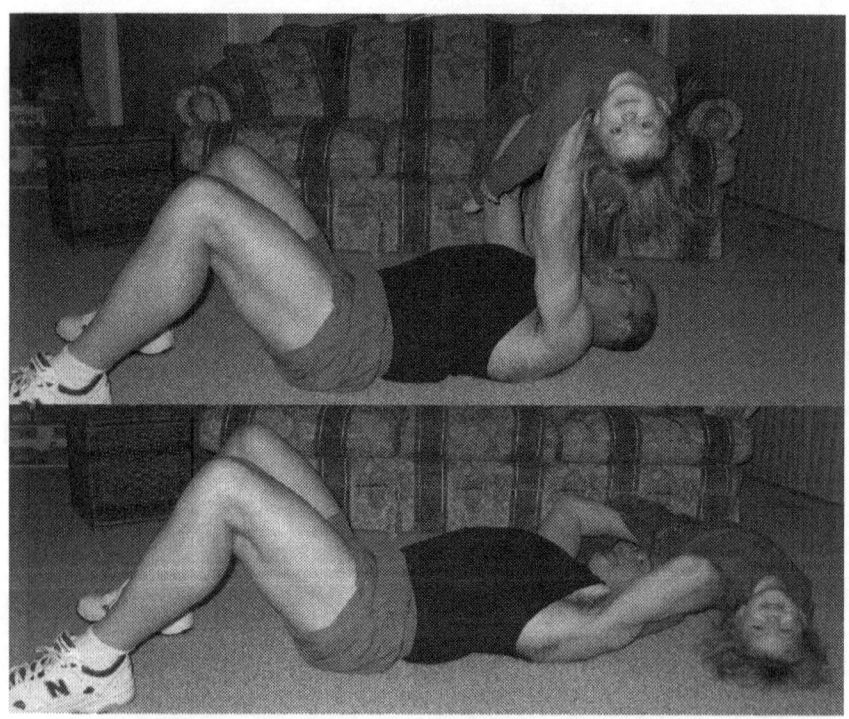

Shoulder Roll

Shoulders & Upper Back

- Have your child stand in front of you.
- Reach under the arms and lock your hands together.
- Raise your shoulders, rotating them from front to back.
- Return to the starting position and do again until the repetition goal is met.

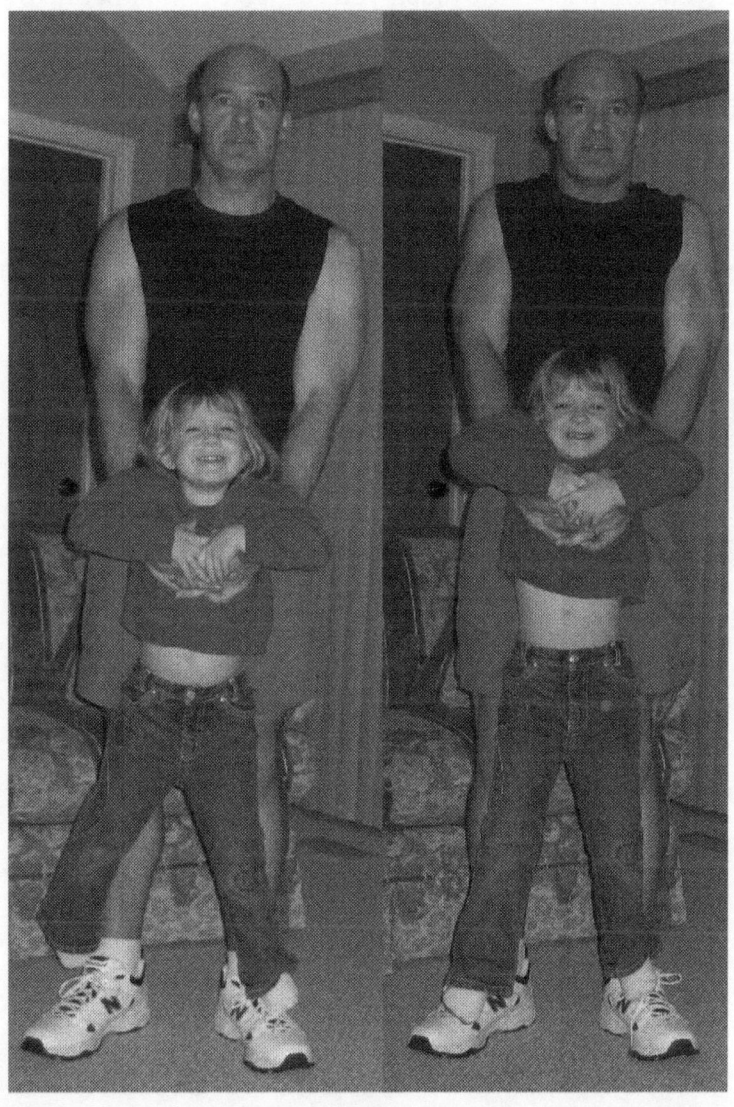

Kid Stretch

Arms

- Have your child stand in front of you with arms in the air.
- Grab him or her by the hands and lift as high as you can.
- Be sure to not jerk your child or pull on one arm. This is an exercise that I have been advised not to perform with my youngest because he has looser joints then a typical child.
- If your child is a little older, you can have him or her help you by jumping.
- Return to the starting position and continue until the repetition goal is met.

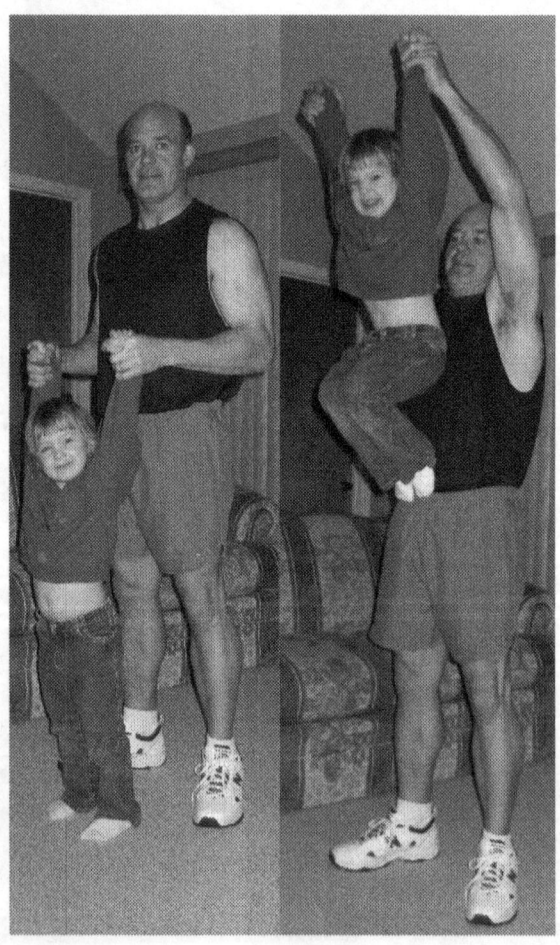

Playground Dips

Arms

- Go to the playground with your kids and find a set of bars that you can suspend yourself in the upright position.
- Lower yourself, keeping your elbows inside.
- Return to the starting position and repeat until desired repetitions are done.

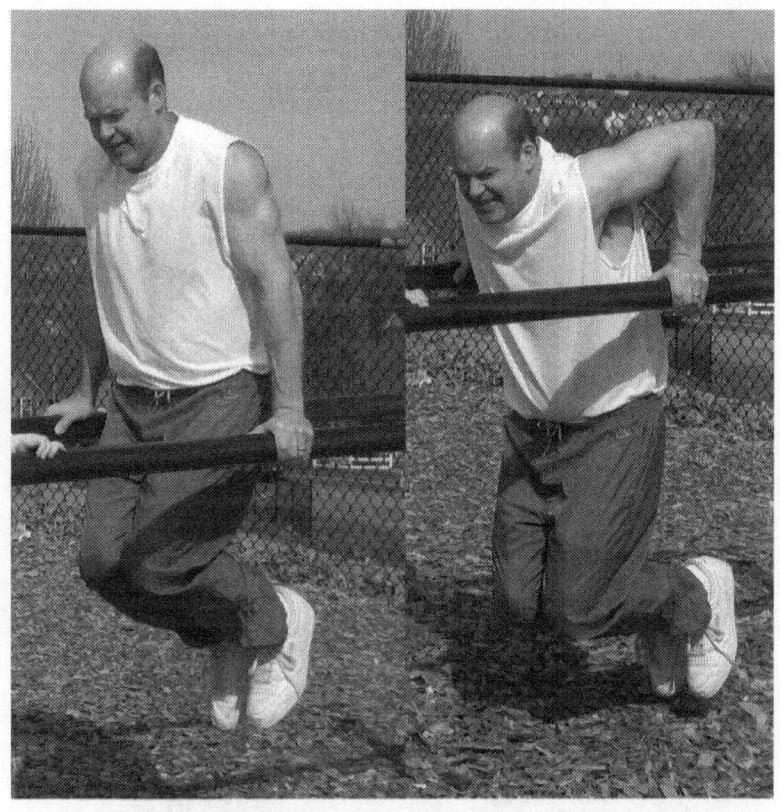

Playground Chin Ups

Back and Arms

- Go to the playground with your kids and find a bar you can hang from.
- Hang from the bar.
- Pull yourself up, trying to touch your chin on the bar.
- Return to the starting position and continue until desired repetitions are met.
- Don't forget to keep an eye on your kids.

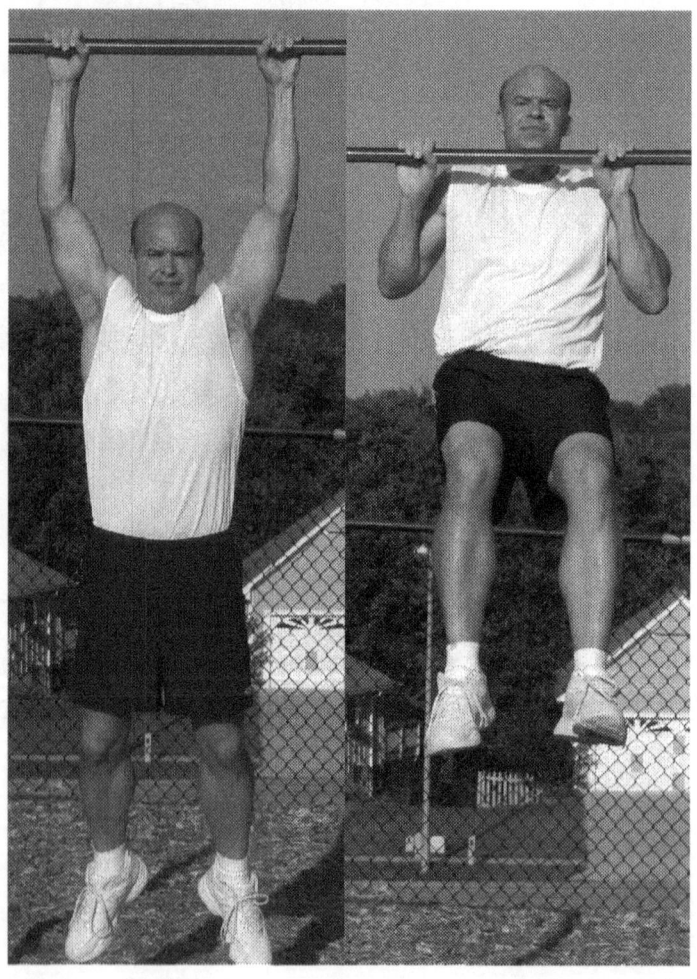

Playground Reverse Chin Ups

Back and Arms

- Go to the playground with your kids and find a bar that you can hang from.
- Hang from the bar with your hands about six inches apart.
- Raise yourself, trying to touch your chin on the bar.
- Return to the starting position. Repeat until desired repetitions are accomplished.

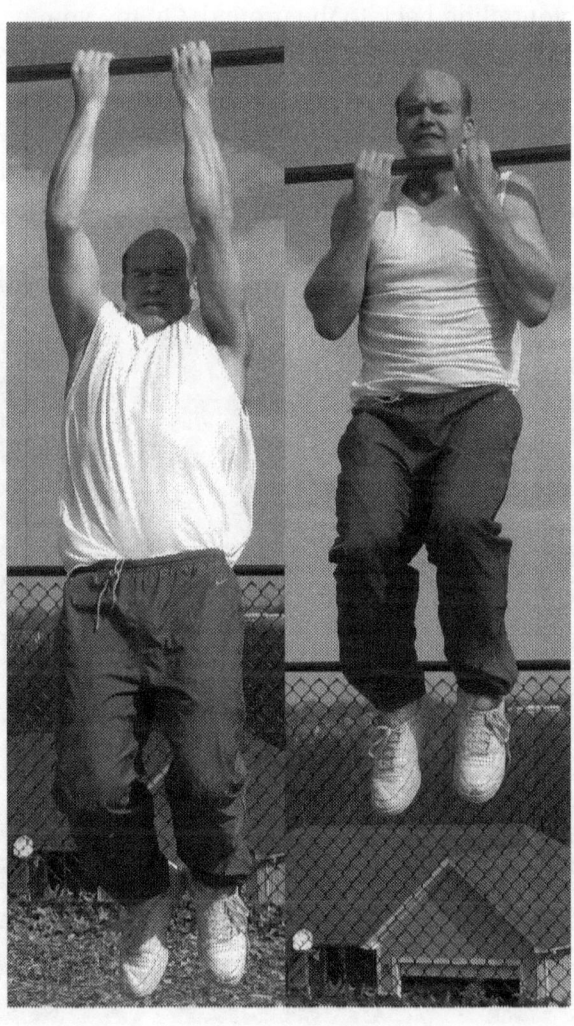

Whole Body Exercises

Rocket

Leg and Arms

- Squat down and place your hands under your child's arms.
- Keep your back as straight as possible.
- Lift your child up into the air as high as you can. ****Do not throw your child into the air.**
- Lower your child back to the ground. On my youngest son, I do not let him touch. On my older children, I let them touch and sometimes allow them to jump to help me. However you do it, be sure your child does not come down on the floor very hard.
- Continue raising and lowering your child in a continuous motion until your repetition goal is achieved.

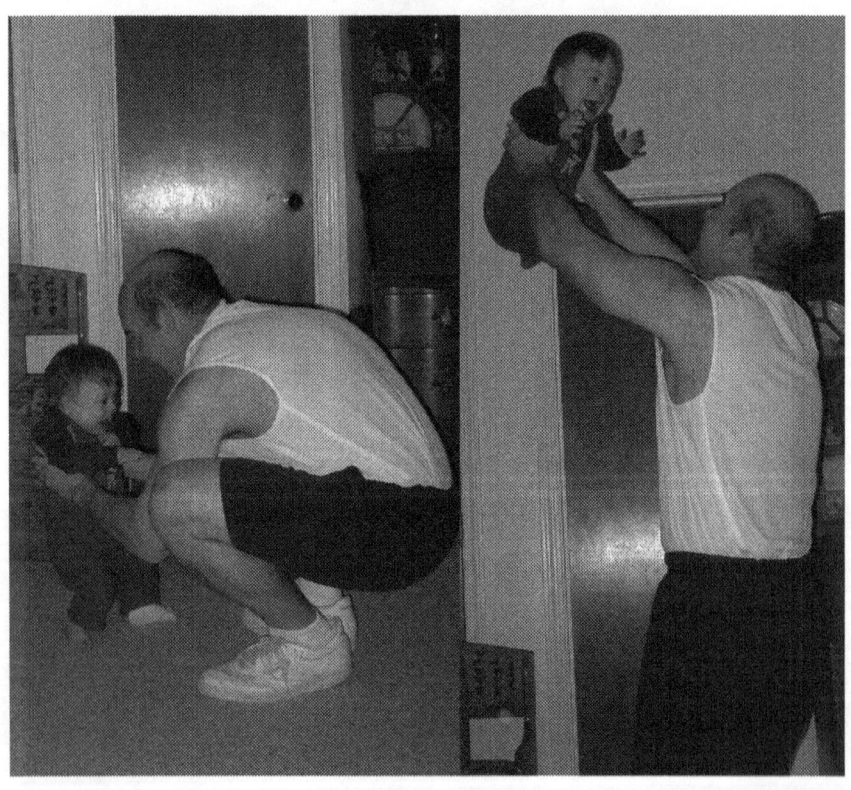

Airplane Squat

Leg and Arms

- This exercise works best with smaller children.
- Place one hand under your child's chest and the other hand under the outside leg.
- Squat down, keeping your back as straight as possible.
- Raise your child as high as is comfortable. ****Do not throw your child in the air.**
- Lower your child.
- Continue raising and lowering in a continuous motion until your repetition goal is achieved.

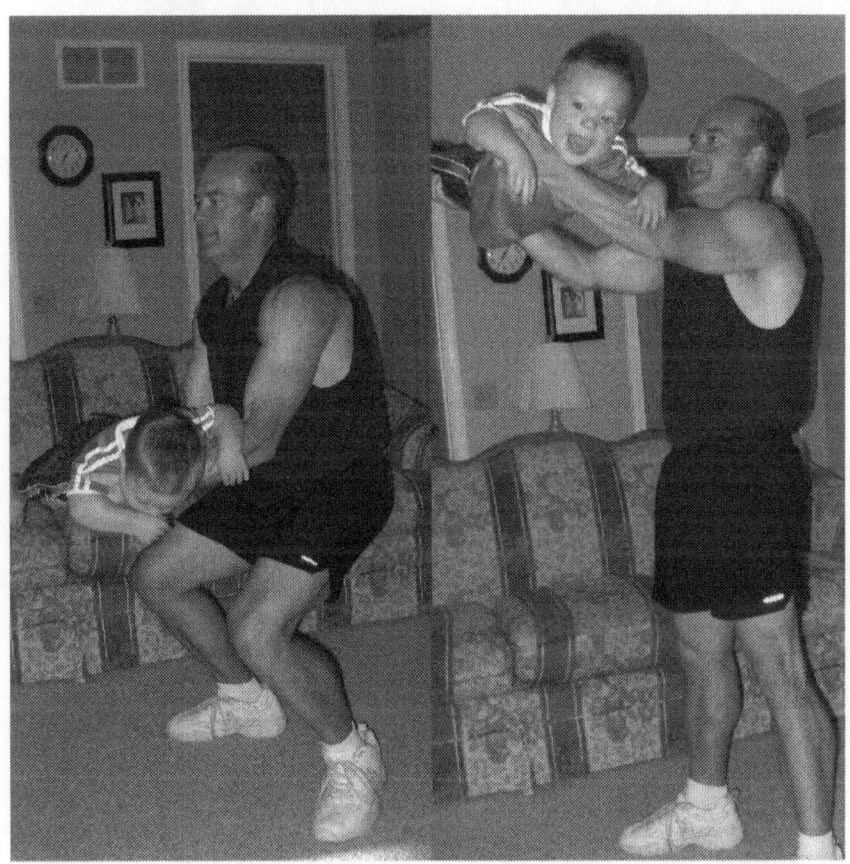

Sit up

Stomach

- Lie with your back on the floor.
- I like to put my toes under the couch keep them from coming up. You can have one of your children sit on your feet to get them involved. If you do use one of your children, don't plan on him or her lasting the whole time.
- Place your hands beside your head.
- Raise yourself until your elbows reach your knees.
- Continue doing sit ups until you reach your repetition goal.

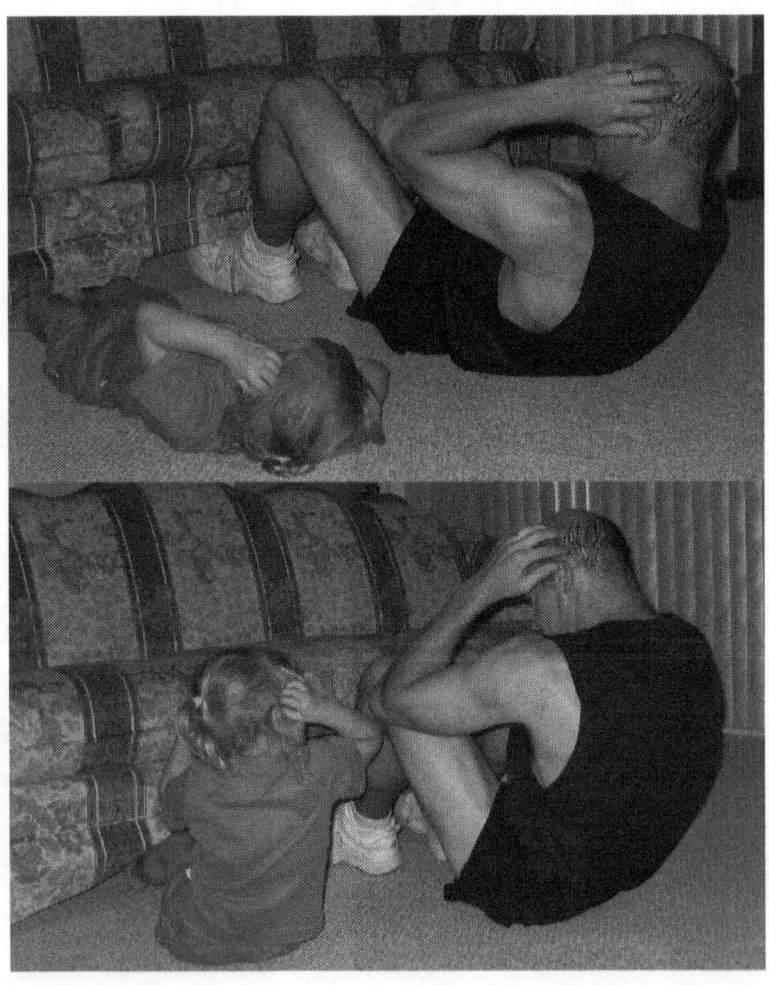

Kid Sit Up

Stomach

- Lie with your back on the floor.
- Place your feet under something like a couch that will keep your feet from coming up.
- Have your child lay himself or herself on your chest with his or her back against your chest.
- Hold onto your child and raise yourself up to a sitting position.
- Continue until your repetition goal is achieved.

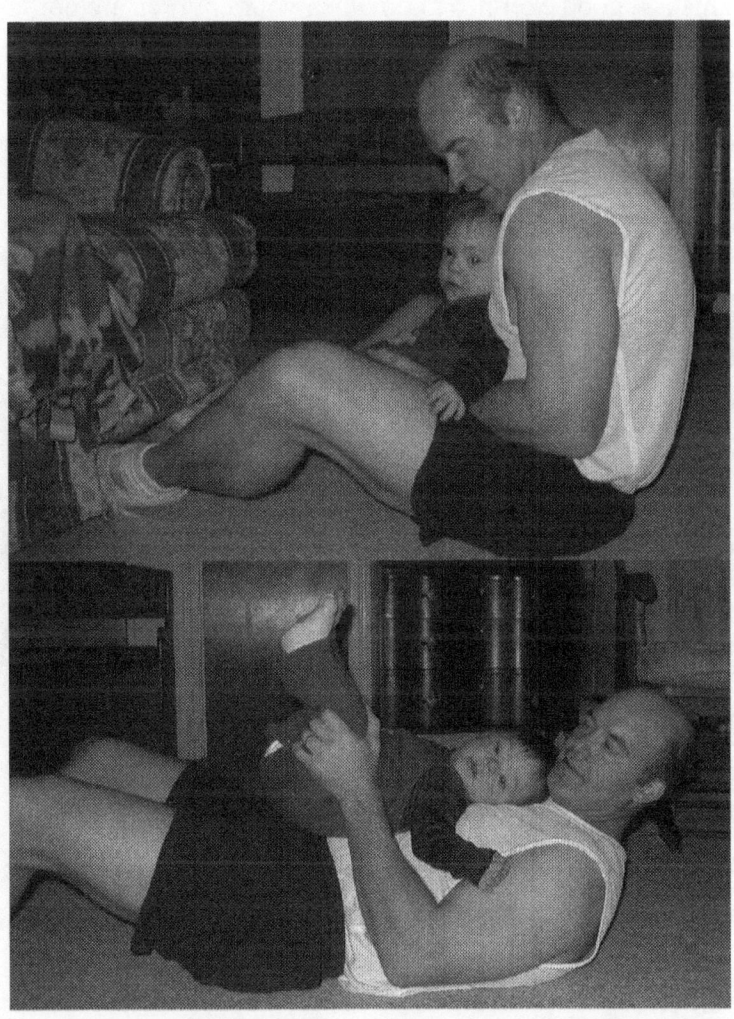

The Crunch

Stomach

- Lie with your back on the floor.
- Raise your legs to somewhere between a 45 to 90 degree angle.
- With your hands beside your head, raise yourself up, concentrating on tightening your stomach muscles.
- Keep your lower back on the floor.
- Hold this position for about five seconds then rest for a couple seconds and go again until your repetition goal is achieved.
- This is a good exercise to do when your children are not available or distracted. My youngest likes to crawl on me while I do these.

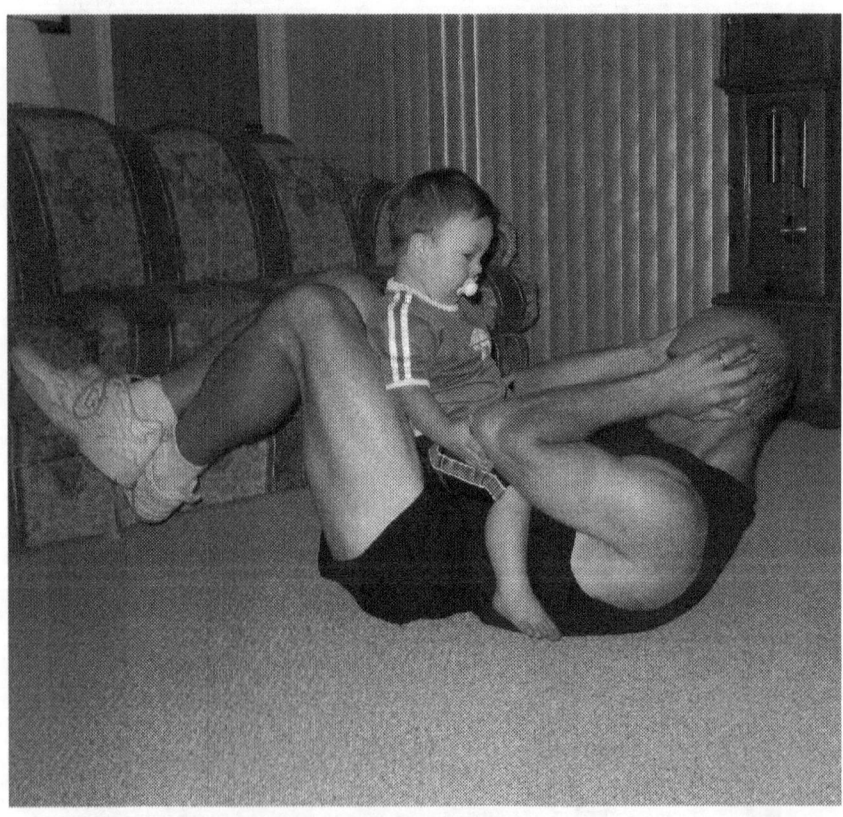

Ultimate Crunch

Stomach

- Lie with your back on the floor.
- Raise your legs to somewhere between a 45 to 90 degree angle.
- Have your child lay on your legs, leaning back over your knees.
- With your hands beside your head, raise shoulders and head, concentrating on tightening your stomach muscles.
- Keep your lower back on the floor.
- Hold this position for about five seconds, then rest for a couple seconds and go again until your repetition goal is achieved.

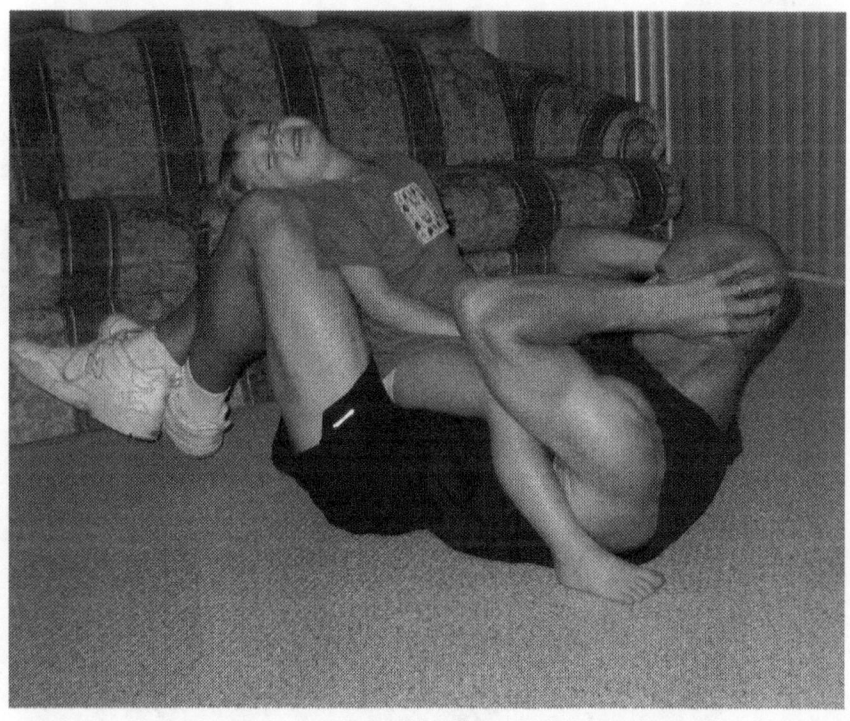

Bounces

Stomach

- Lie with your back on the floor.
- Have your smaller child sit on your stomach.
- Support them either by holding their hands or their body.
- Raise your derriere up and down making your child bounce on your stomach. Don't move up and down more then two or three inches and don't be too rough.
- Keep your back on the floor.
- Lower your head to feel a different workout.
- Continue to bounce until either you or your child is ready to move on.
- This was an exercise that my youngest son could participate in very early. It helped include him when he was too young for most of the other exercises.

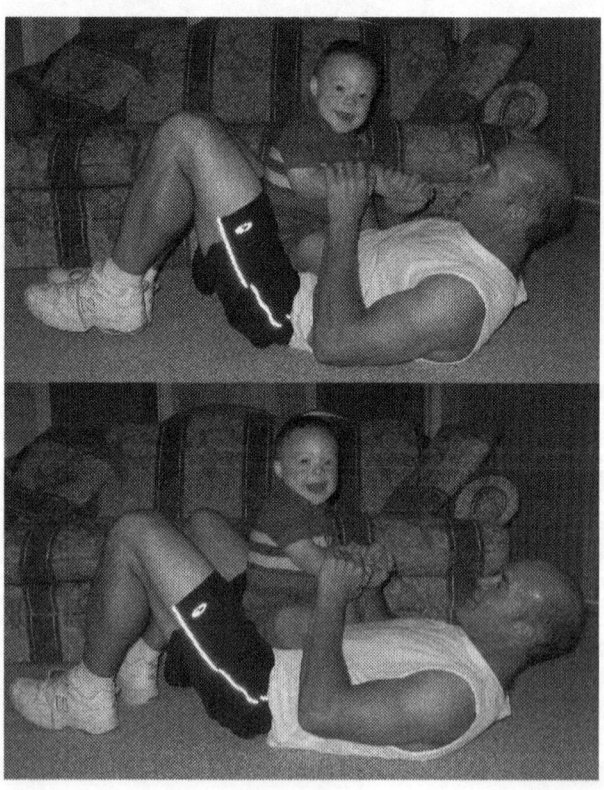

Rock, Paper, Scissors

Stomach and Legs

- Lie with your back to the floor, your hands under your derriere.
- Raise your knees, keeping your feet off the floor.
- Keep your lower back on the floor.
- Lower your head to feel a different workout.
- Extend your legs, keeping your feet about six inches off the floor.
- Spread your legs apart, still keeping them about six inches off the floor.
- Bring your legs back to the straight position.
- Return them to the starting position and continue until repetition goal is achieved.

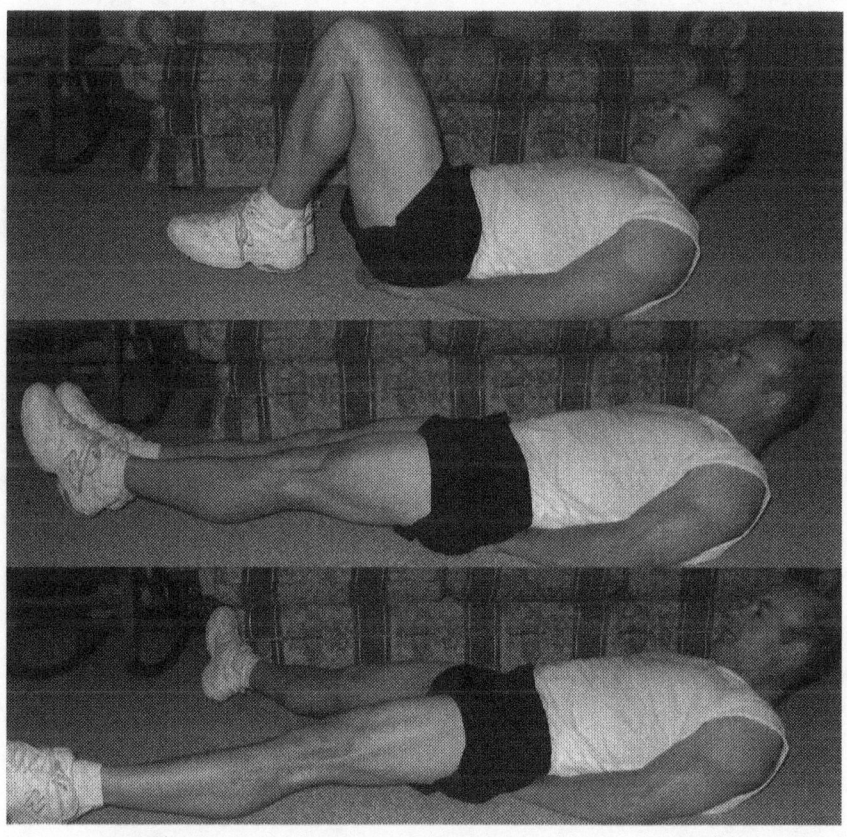

Loader

Stomach and Legs

- Lie with your back on the floor and have your child sit on your stomach.
- Raise your knees, keeping your feet off the floor.
- Keep your lower back on the floor.
- Grab your child under the legs, being sure you have a good grip. If you do not feel secure holding your child this way you can grab them under their arms.
- Extend your legs, keeping your feet about six inches off the floor, and lift your child into the air.
- Bring your legs back to the straight position and lower your child back to your chest.
- Continue the exercise until you reach your repetition goal.

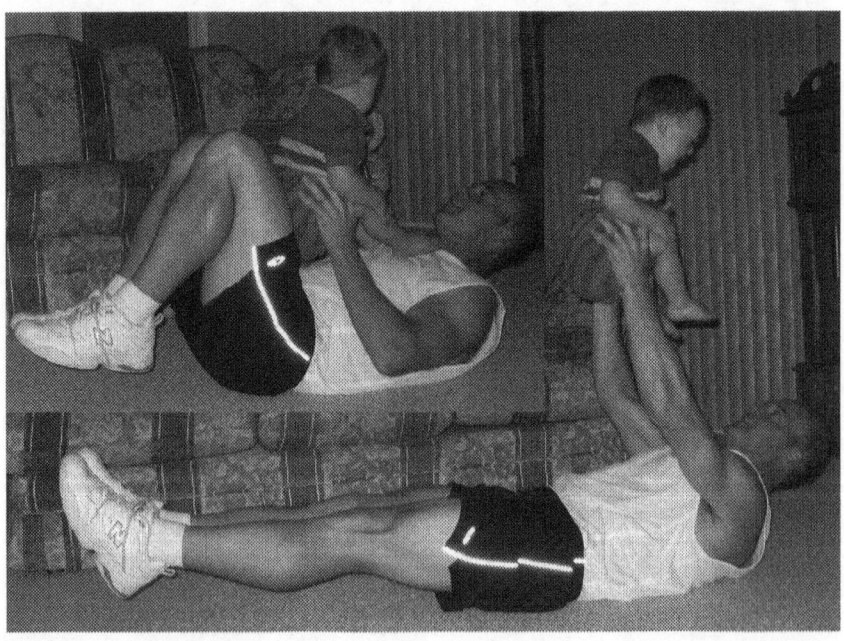

The Perch

Stomach

- Lie with your back on the floor, your derriere almost against the wall, and your legs up the wall.
- Pick your wall space carefully. DADsercise can be dangerous if you cross Mom by marking up the wall.
- Flex your knees and have your child sit on your feet.
- Raise your legs back up. Your children really don't add anything to the exercise, but they sure seem to have fun sitting on their high perch.
- With your hands beside your head, raise yourself, concentrating on tightening the stomach muscles.
- Hold this position for about five seconds, then rest for a couple seconds and go again until you achieve the repetition goal.

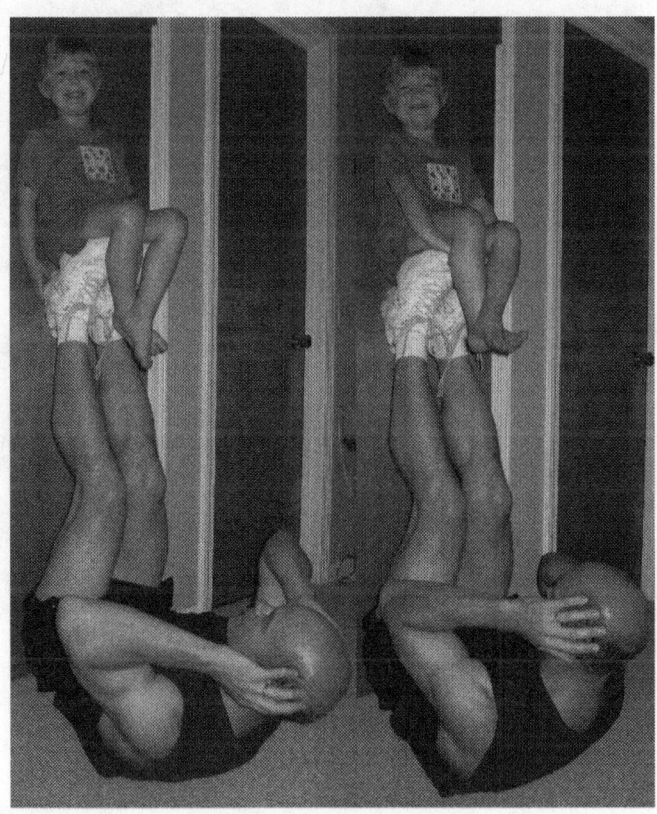

Side Leans

Stomach – Love Handles (side torso)

- Lift your child onto your shoulders.
- Lean to the left and hold for a second.
- Contract your abs while bending.
- Straighten back up.
- Lean to the right and hold for a second.
- Straighten back up and continue until the repetition goal is met.
- ****Do not lean so far that you become overbalanced.**

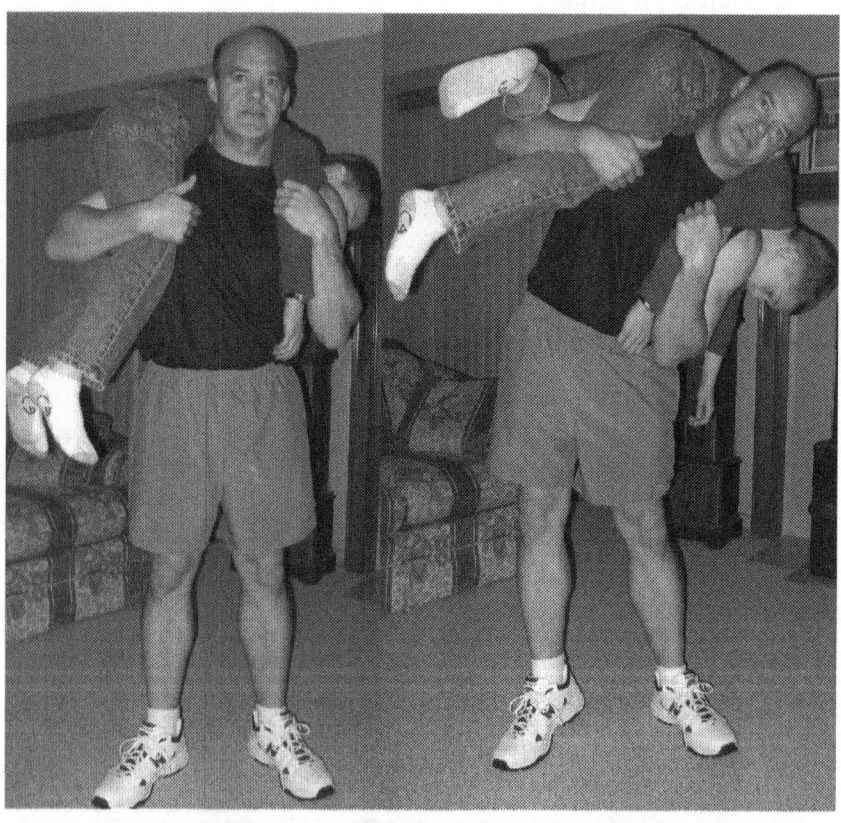

Helicopter

Stomach – Love Handles (side torso)

- Lift your child up on your shoulders.
- Sit down on a chair with a low back.
- Twist your upper body to the left.
- Contract your abs while bending.
- Twist back to the right and repeat until repetition goal is met.
- When done, stand up and set your child down.

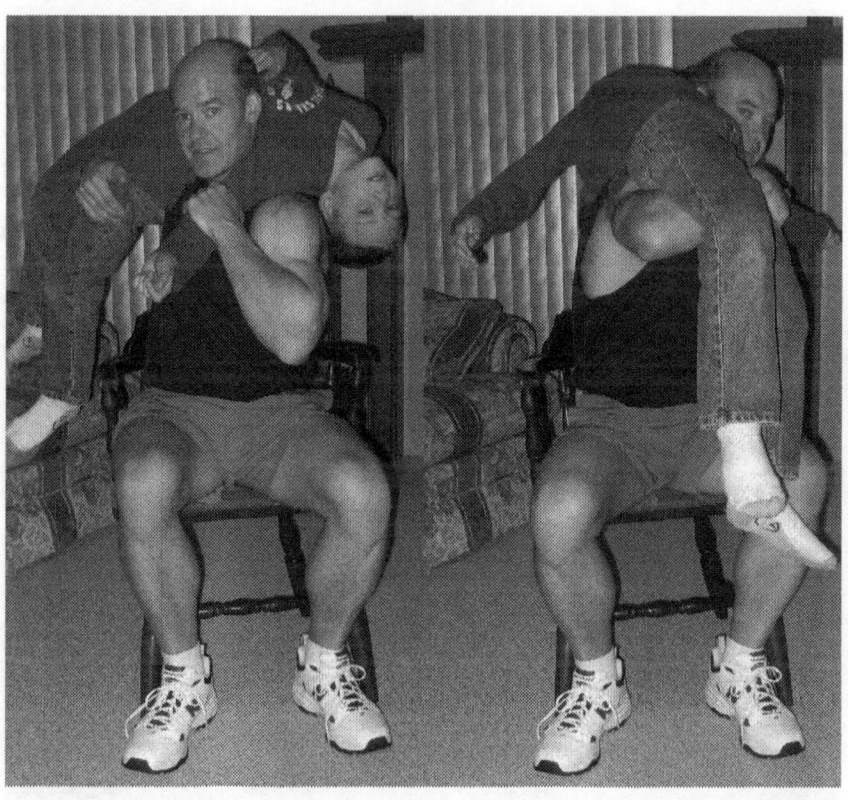

Couch Butt Raises

Stomach

- Lie on your back with your feet on a couch.
- Have your child sit on your stomach.
- Raise your derriere off the ground.
- Lower it to the ground and repeat until repetitions are done.
- Relax and lower your head for a different workout.
- (Optional) Make goofy sounds to make it more fun.

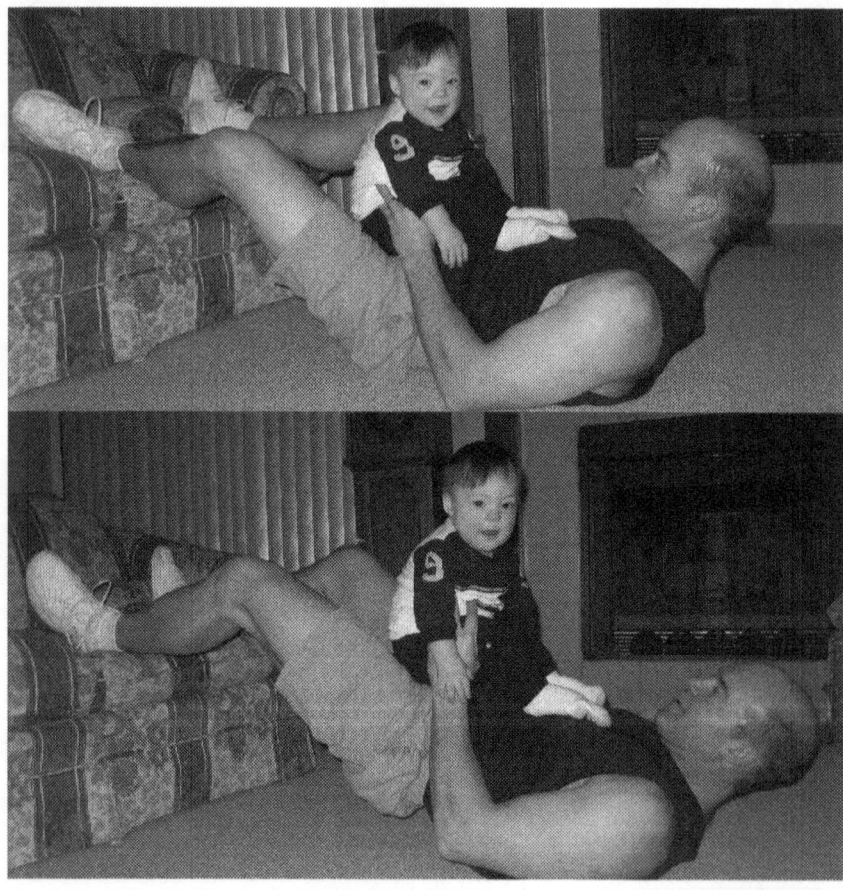

Playground Leg Raises

Stomach

- Go to the playground with your children.
- Find some bars that are parallel from the ground. You might have trouble finding this equipment. I don't find bars at every playground.
- Suspend yourself above the ground with your body in a straight position.
- Raise your legs as high as you can and hold for a few seconds.
- Lower your legs continuing to suspend yourself.
- Do as many as you can, then rest and do another set

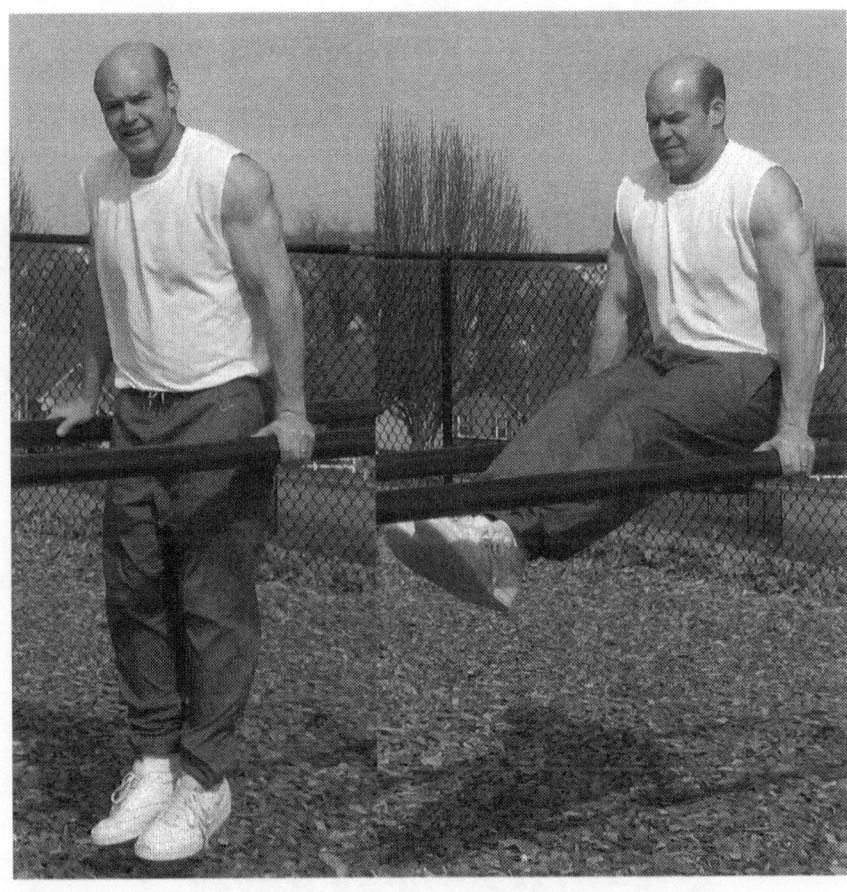

Hanging Crossover

Stomach and Side Torso

- Go to the playground with your kids.
- Find a sturdy bar that can hold you.
- Hang from the bar.
- Raise your knees, bringing them over to one side and hold for several seconds.
- Lower your legs.
- Raise your knees, bringing them over to the opposite side, and hold for several seconds.
- Continue until the repetition goal is met.

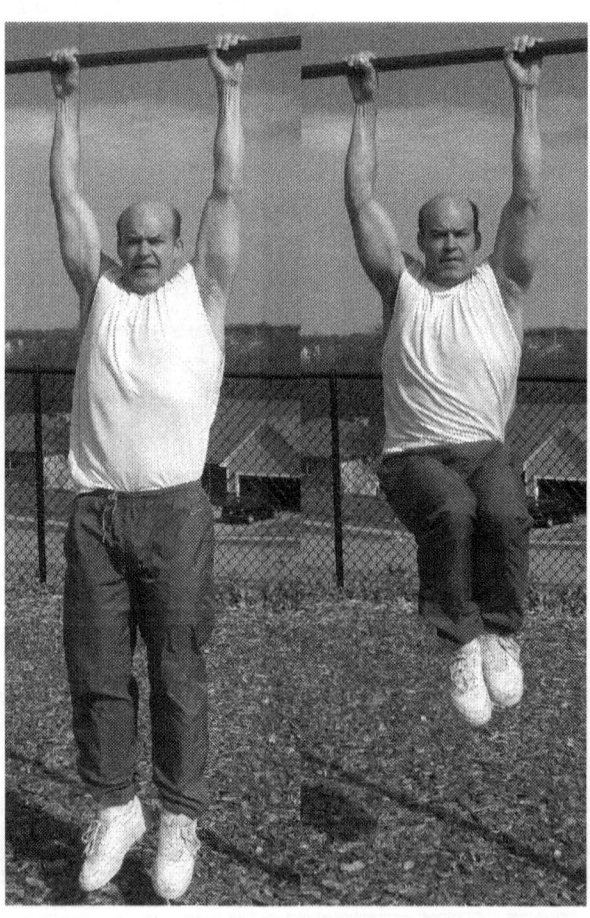

Lower Body Exercises

Squat

Legs

- Lift your child up and place him or her on your shoulders. I find having my child lie across my shoulders much safer than having him or her sit on my shoulders.
- Bend your knees, lowering yourself toward to the ground and keeping your back straight.
- Straighten yourself back up and repeat until the desired repetitions are done.
- Be sure to be in a standing position when you set your child down.

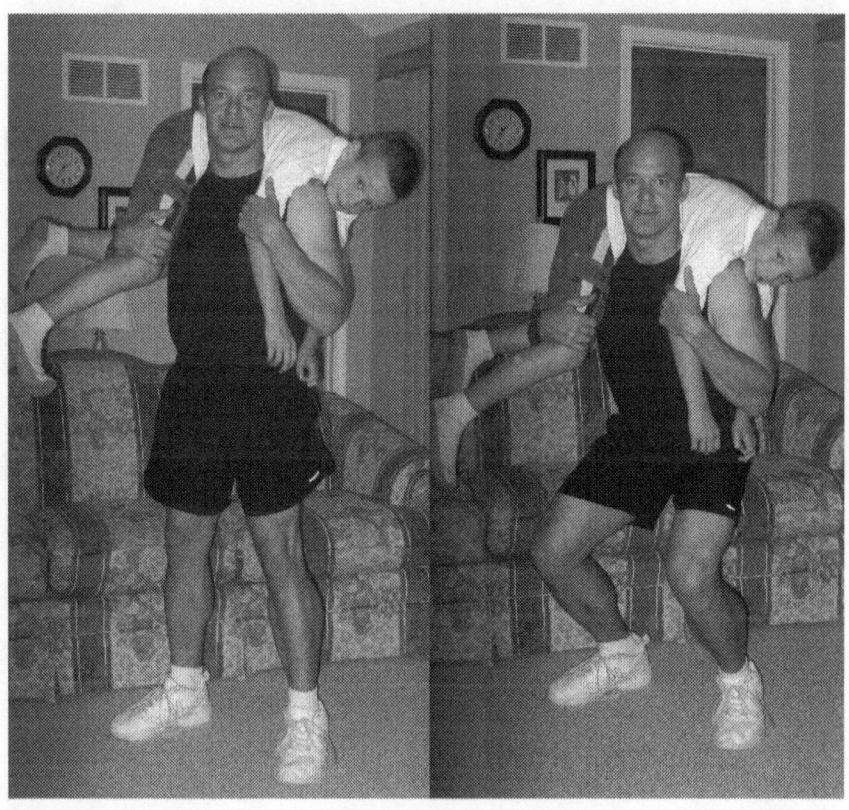

Front Lunge

Upper Legs

- Hold your smaller child in your arms in front of you.
- Extend one leg in front of you.
- Lean forward, bending your extended leg.
- Be careful not to extend your front knee past your toes to avoid strain to the knee.
- Raise yourself back up and repeat.
- Switch legs and do again until the repetition goal is met.

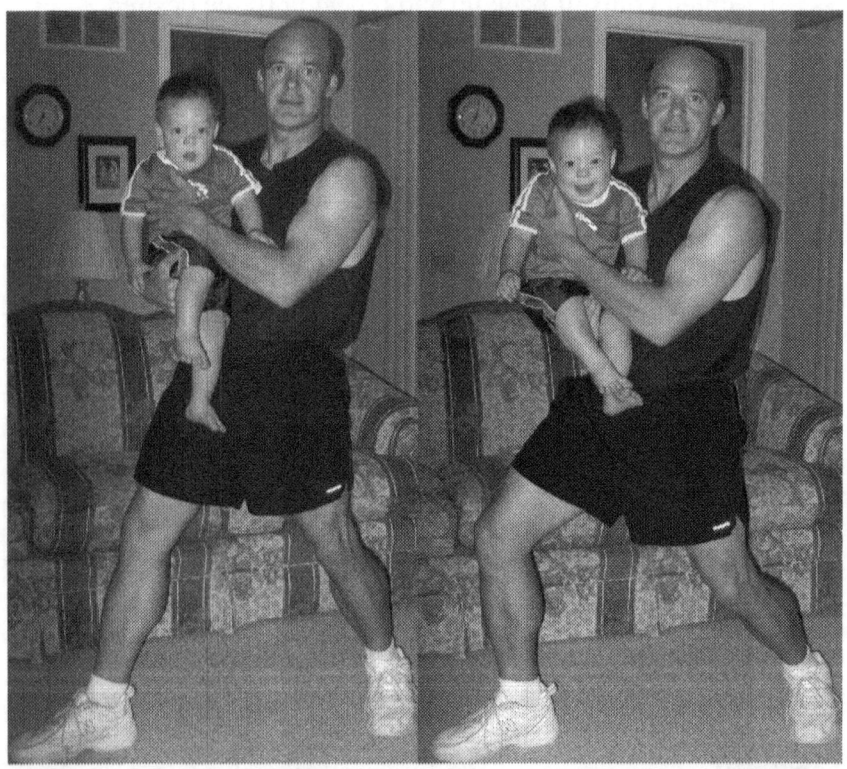

Side Lunge

Upper Legs

- Hold your smallest child in your arms in front of you.
- Extend one leg out to one side.
- Lean sideways, bending your extended leg.
- Be careful not to extend your front knee past your toes to avoid strain to the knee.
- Raise yourself back up and repeat.
- Switch legs and do again until repetition goal is met.

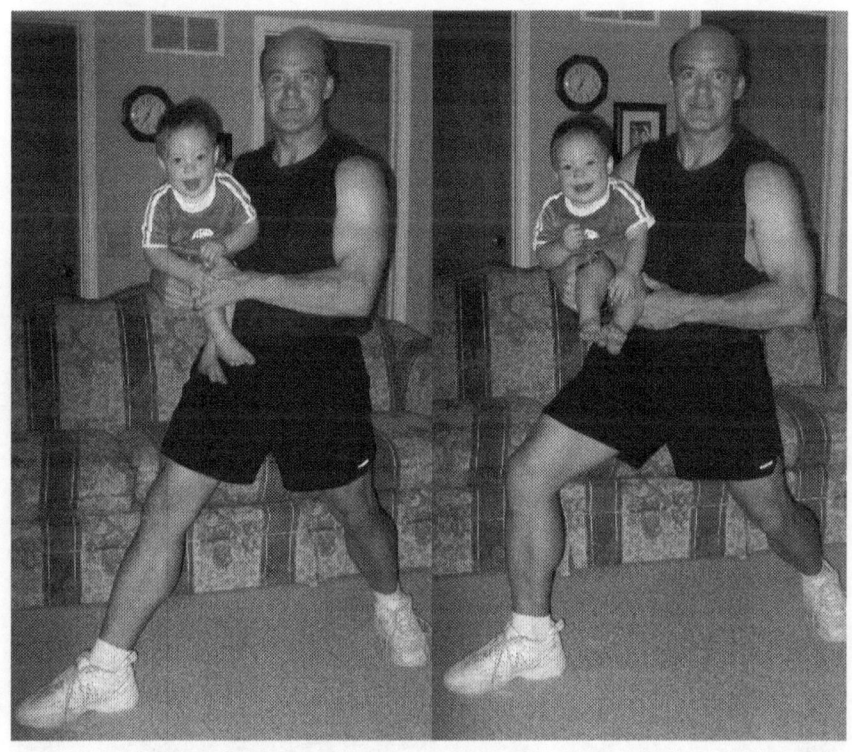

Reverse Leg Lift

Upper Leg

- Grab a pillow or a couch cushion
- Lie on the floor with your feet on the couch and your chest on the pillow.
- Have your child sit on your legs with his or her derriere right on the back of your knees.
- Straighten your legs, lifting your child.
- Lower your legs and continue until the repetition goal is met.

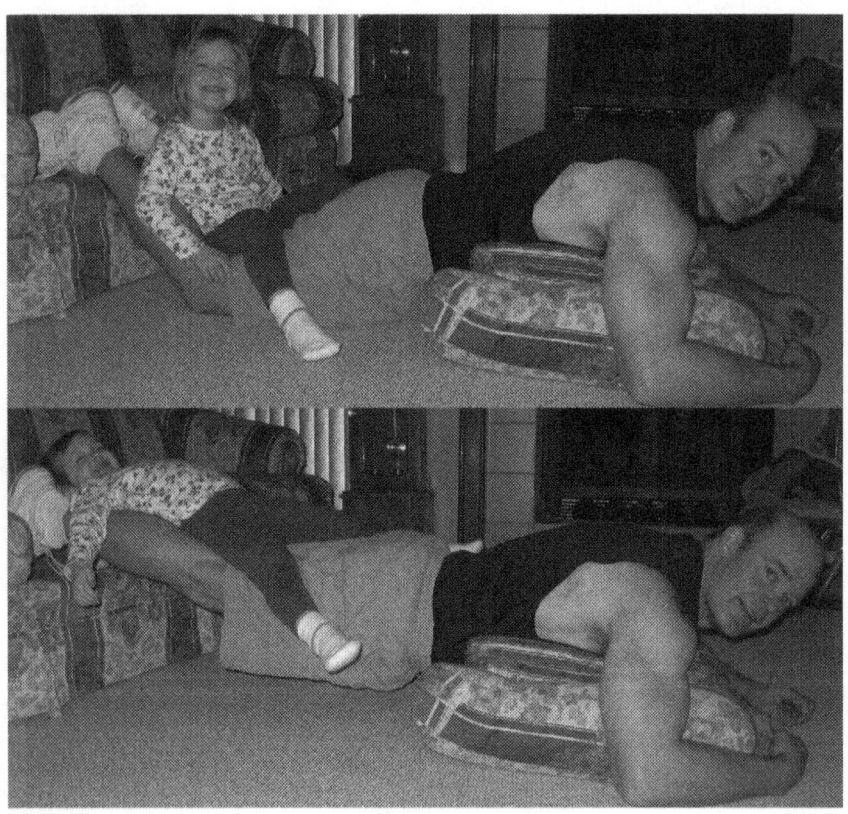

Front Leg Lift

Legs and Stomach

- Lie on the floor with your knees in the air.
- Have your child sit on the top of your feet and hang on to the hands.
- Straighten your legs, lifting your child up into the air.
- Lower your legs and continue until repetition goal is met.

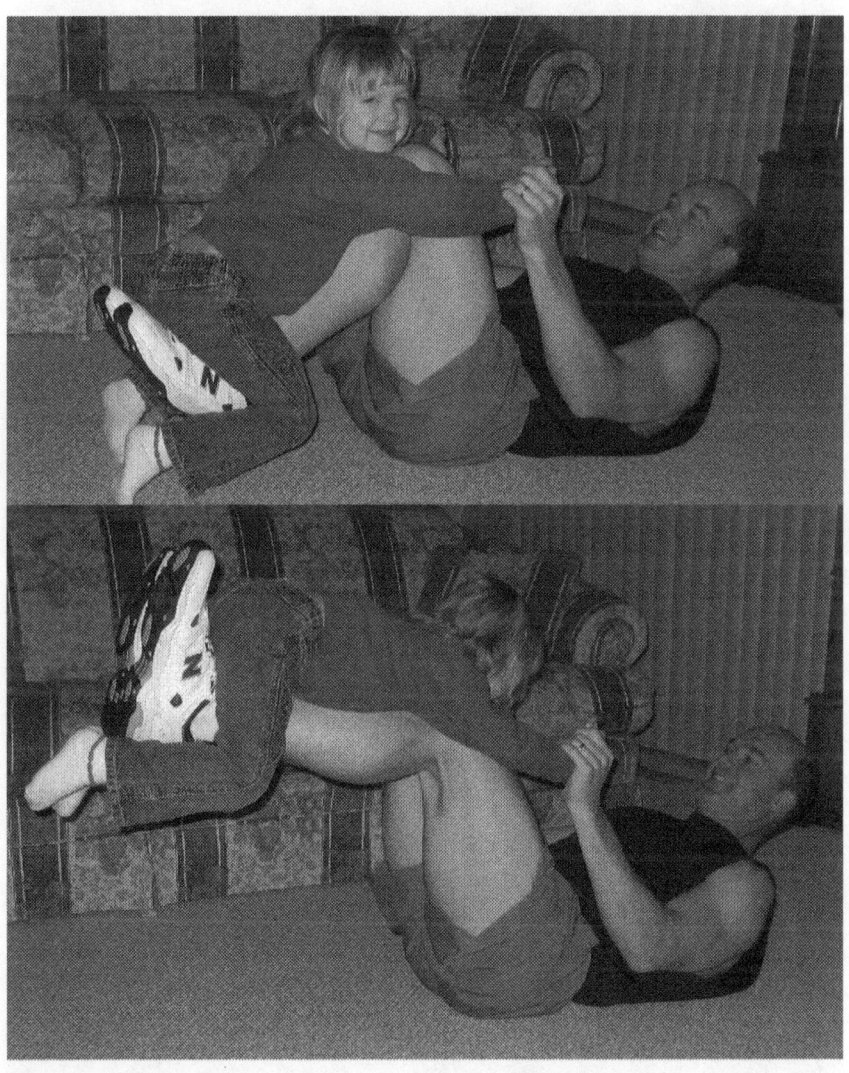

Calf Raises

Lower Leg (calves)

- Lift your child onto your shoulders
- Place your toes on something like a thick book.
- Raise your heels off the ground.
- Lower your heels and continue until the repetition goal is met.

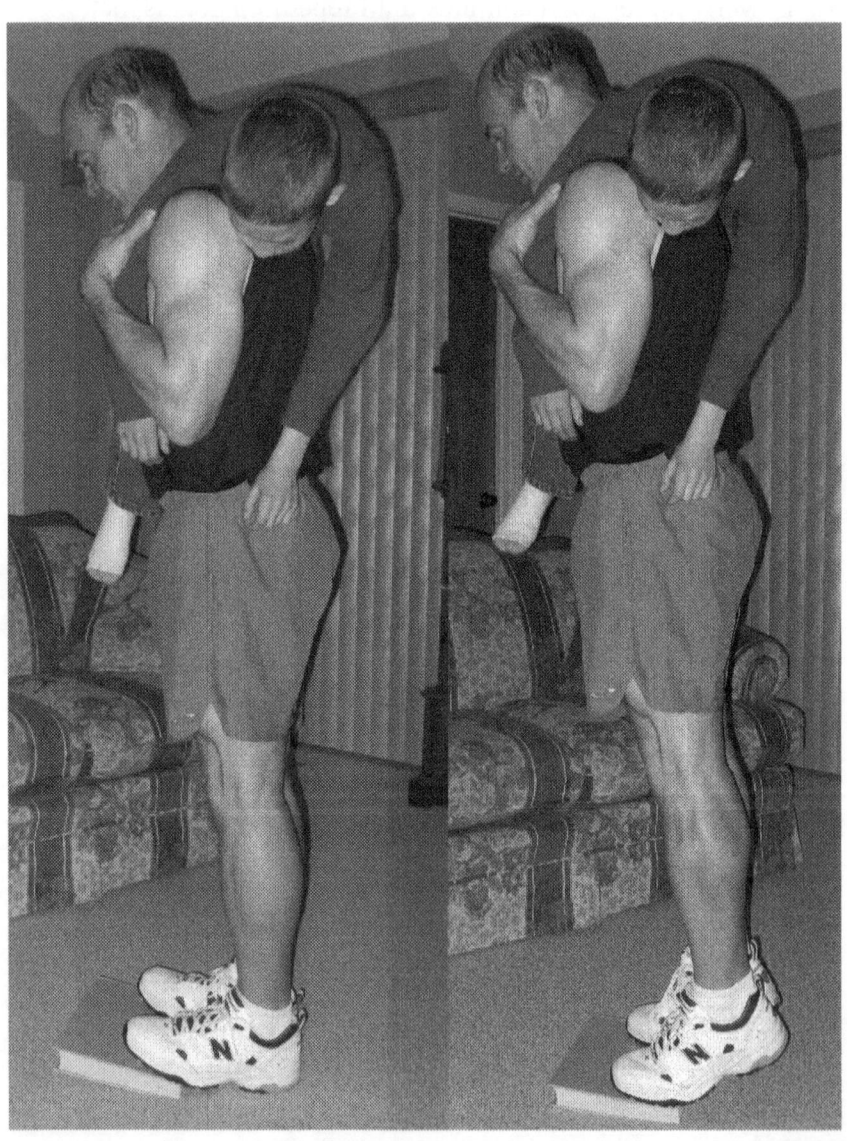

Reverse Leg Raises

Upper Leg (hamstring)

- Lie on your stomach on the floor.
- Have your child lie on your legs with their derriere on the back of your knees. My children like to bring a pillow for the head.
- Bend your legs, raising your child.
- Lower your legs and continue until the repetition goal is met.

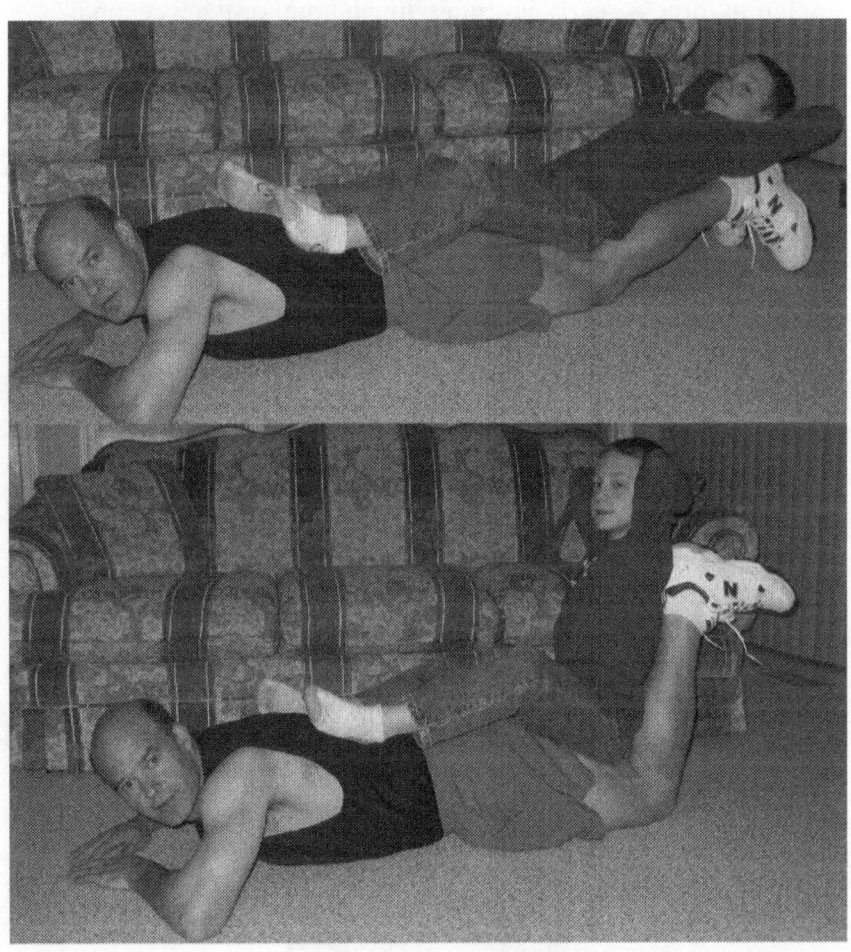

Cardiovascular

Although most of the DADsercise exercises focus on building skeletal muscle mass, the most important muscle in the body is the heart. As I have mentioned several times, getting a good cardiovascular workout is a crucial component of DADsercise. I get most of my cardiovascular workout by running either outside or on a treadmill. I try to slip this activity in when it won't affect my family time — early morning, lunch hour, or the weekend.

I realize running may not be your thing. I suggest, however, finding a good cardiovascular workout that fits your style. Even though it wasn't high on the priority list at the start of my DADsercise experience, running now comprises most of my heart work exercises. Here are a few other ways that I found to get the ol' heart pumping.

Popcorn

This one is very simple. Hold hands with your child and then jump up and down together. If you have several children, have them line up and take turns. My daughter loves to do this. Be sure to not jerk your child or pull on one arm.

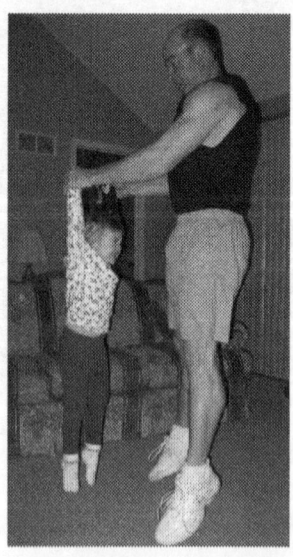

Living Room Motion

Living Room Motion is a variation of a workout that my son's wrestling team does. Since our living room is a bit smaller than the gym, things had to be altered a bit. Performed over a period of time, this is a good multi-exercise workout that can be done with your older kids.

***Find a room where you and your kids can move back and forth 10 to 15 feet. You will also need a clock or a timer of some sort.

Living Room Motion Steps

1. Jog for 30 seconds
2. Skip High for 30 seconds
3. 20 Pushups
4. 20 Sit-ups
5. 20 Jumping Jacks
6. Jog for 30 seconds
7. Shuffle for 30 seconds
8. 5 Foot Fires & Sprawls
9. 10 Jacks Jumps

*Repeat until desired repetitions are done

1. Jog

Jogging in the living room needs to be a little different than when jogging outside. You need to combine jogging in place with jogging so you don't move across the room very fast.

2. Skip High

Skip High is pretty much what it sounds like. Skip across the room, bringing your knees up to parallel. Again, you don't want to move across the room too fast, so try to move vertically more than horizontally.

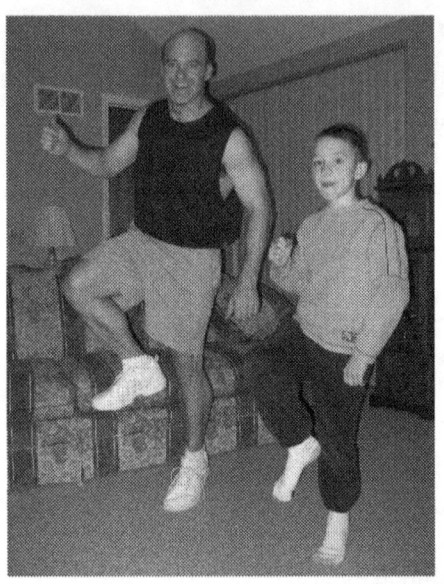

3. Pushup

Pick your method of pushup. I typically just do the standard pushup.

4. Sit up

Again, I typically do a standard sit up.

5. Jumping Jacks

Nothing fancy here. Just a standard jumping jack.

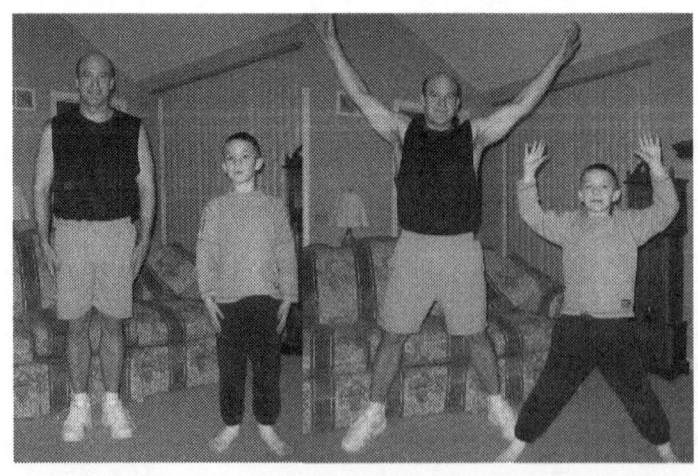

6. Jog

7. Shuffle

The shuffle is a way of moving across the floor sideways. This is important for wrestlers to stay in good position around the mat while facing the opponent. Even if you are not one of those dads who is training for one of the Old Timers Wrestling meets, this is a really good exercise.

Squat down, keeping fairly low. Go sideways, moving the leading foot in the direction you want to move and then bring the following foot next to the lead foot. Continue in the direction until you get to the end of the room and then go back the other direction.

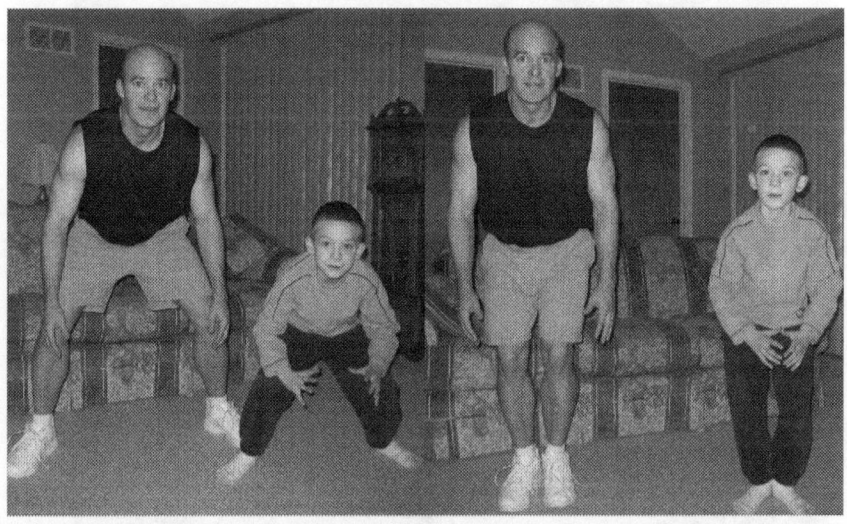

8. Foot Fire & Sprawl

Be sure that you have stretched your arms and shoulders well before doing this exercise. Two years ago I showed my son a version of this exercise; I still feel a twinge every once in a while in my shoulder. I guess I don't get over things as fast as I used to.

This exercise has two parts. The first part is running in place as fast as you can while taking small steps. You should look like your feet are on fire. Continue to do the Foot Fire for about 5 seconds and then call out "Sprawl." Drop your chest to the floor and then get up as fast as you can to return to the Foot Fire. Your kids will have fun doing this one with you. See who can get up the fastest.

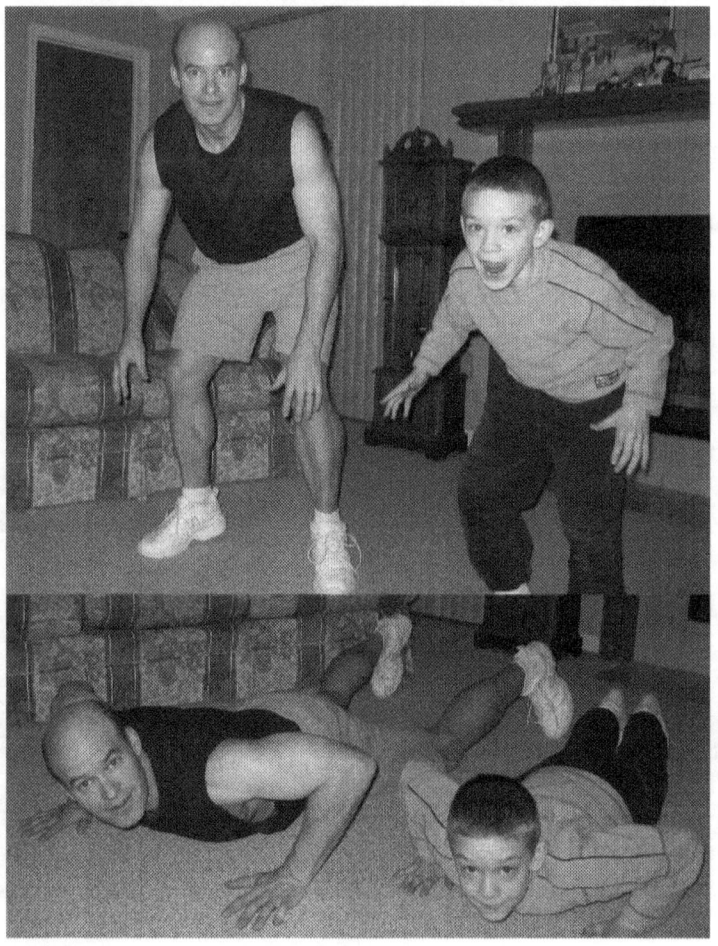

9. Jack Jumps
A Jack Jump is simply jumping in the air, bringing your knees up as high as you can.

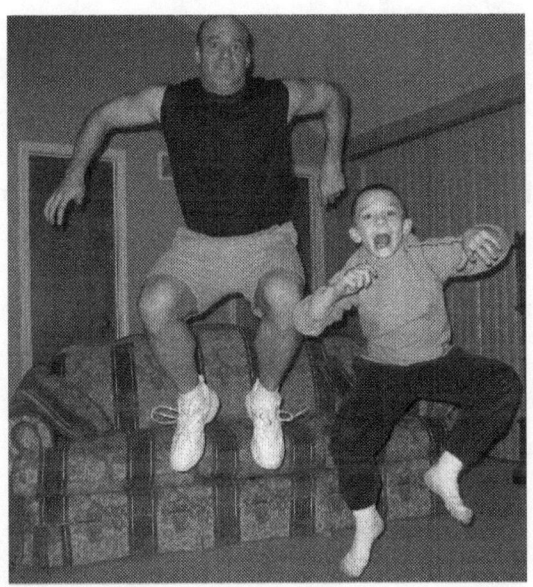

Alternative Living room Motion

If your living room does not have enough space to do the living room motion. You can come up with some alternate plans. My son and I have altered it by doing 30 pushups, 30 sit ups, 30 jumping jacks, 5 foot fires & sprawls, and then 10 jack jumps. This compresses the workout, making the jumping jacks the rest time instead of the jogging.

Stairs

Good old stairs. My fondest memories of running stairs were my freshman year at state wrestling in Lincoln, Nebraska. At that time if you lost your first match, you had to wait to see if the person who beat you won his next match. I had gotten beat by a fellow freshman, who was to face a senior next. I was sure he was going to get beat, and I would be done. A few hours later the freshman won; I remember setting down my unfinished ice cream cup to go weigh myself. I was four pounds over the legal weight limit. By morning, I was still two pounds over. That day I touched every step in the arena. The Bob Devaney Sports Center has a lot of steps. I did make weight! I realize now that the weight I lost was mainly water, but what a workout!

Tag Team Stairs

This is a good one to do with that older child who may feel the need to rest frequently. Start at either the top or the bottom of the steps, whichever has the most room. Whoever starts first begins running up the stairs (one at a time preferably) and then walking down the steps. You might want to make the repetitions five times up and down the steps. On your fifth repetition, tag your child and then encourage as he or she runs the steps. Keep going back and forth until you both complete the desired repetitions. Increase the repetitions as you both get into better shape.

Conclusion

One morning as I returned from my morning run, my wife met me at the door, holding my squirming son Daniel. Although sweat was dripping off me, he wanted to jump into my arms. Laughing, Janet and I reflected on how special he was to our family, as are all our children; however, if it wasn't for his coming into our family, I would not have been out running that morning or even thinking about exercising. I thought about how far I had come. My life has changed since Daniel's heart surgery; I hope it doesn't take an event such as the one my family went through to get you inspired.

Getting motivated allowed me to achieve more than I ever expected. I don't have a good "before" picture of me, my belly hanging out, my pants bursting at the seams, like you see in the diet ads. To be honest, I was a little embarrassed about my physique. I doubt I would have wanted to pose for a picture. The real reason, however, that I don't have a good "before" picture is that I never expected such a dramatic change when I first began the "fun."

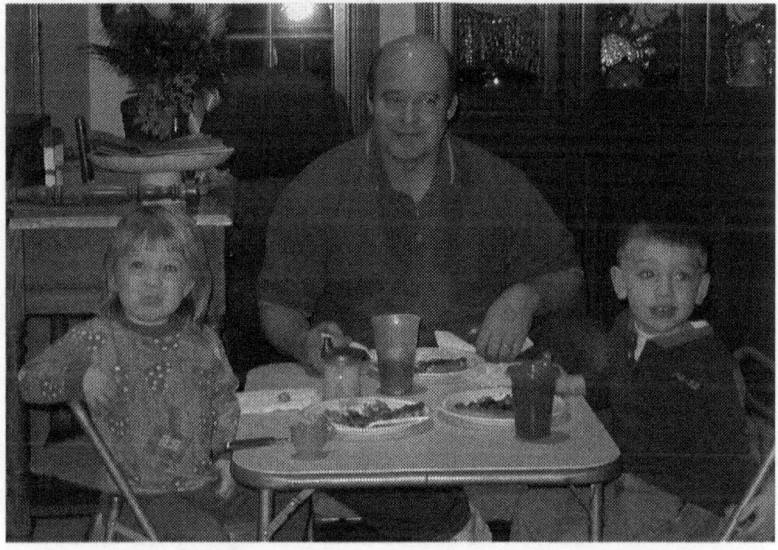

Here is a picture that was taken shortly before I decided to start exercising. I was weighing in around 215 pounds. In the picture I am eating at the kids' table, but obviously I was not eating a kid's portion.

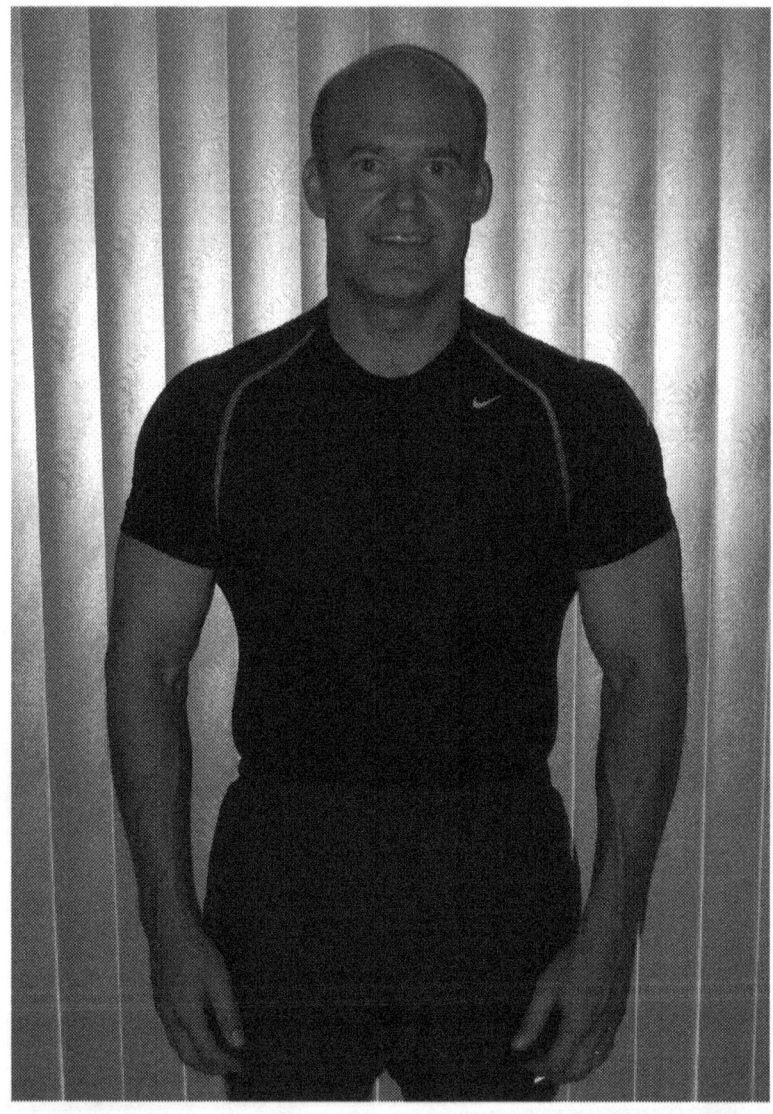

This picture is not nearly as embarrassing. At the time of this picture I weighed about 168 pounds. I have been maintaining this weight for about four months to the time of this writing.

I'm sure it's obvious by the pictures that I not only feel better, I also feel better about myself. I feel more productive at work, and I can actually go to the swimming pool and not worry about the harpoons of whispered remarks. In fact, I enjoy the comments now!

This transformation, however, did not happen overnight. I made a lifestyle change, not a change in diet or pills. I was very patient, continuing to exercise, even when there were worrisome plateaus when I didn't lose weight. I even gained back a few pounds from time to time. It took about seven months for me to lose 45 pounds, going from a 36 inch waist to a 30. In comparison to fad diet claims, this must seem like a horribly slow process. All I can say is - what's the hurry? It took me over ten years to get in poor condition. What are six or seven months to take it off? Let's not forget, I was and am still having fun with my kids. It has been a great family experience and will continue to be. Since I have a one year old, a four year old, and an eight year old, I can see our family dynamics continuing to change. In a few years my oldest will be too big for me to lift while my youngest will be able to participate in exercises that he is unable to today. I'll have to come up with new ways to include all the kids. Is anybody ready for DADsercise II?

Your situation will be different than mine no doubt. Customize an exercise plan that works best for you. Make it part of your daily, weekly, monthly, and yearly routine. Throw the kids into the mix and make some memories!

Have fun! Really!

Appendix

This appendix contains a blank goal chart and a blank workout journal. Feel free to photocopy these pages from the appendix to use them. Since the book's print is not in a letter-sized page, you can find the full-sized version of these documents on the www.dadsercise.com web site.

DADsercise Goal Chart

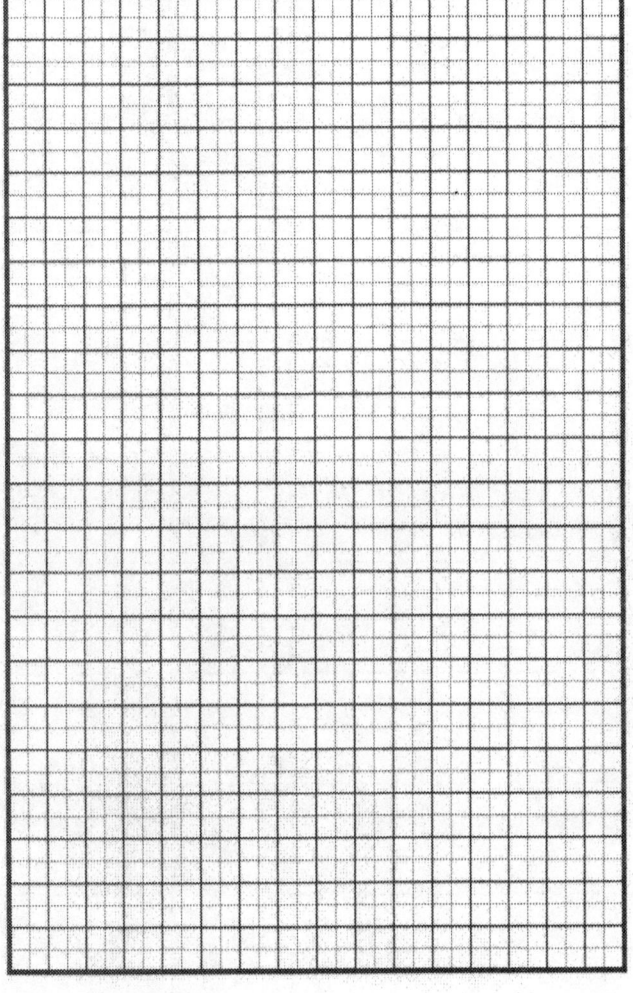

www.dadsercise.com

DADsercise Daily Workout Journal

Day/Date	Exercise	Upper Body	Abs	Legs	Cardio	Set 1		Set 2		Set 3	
						Child	Reps	Child	Reps	Child	Reps

About the Author

Perry Schnacker has lived a life of diversity. Raised on a Central Nebraska farm, he graduated in 1984 as salutatorian of his class and was a top-ranked wrestler in the state for a time. After high school he earned his bachelor's degree in Computer Science at the University of Nebraska at Kearney, his tuition subsidized by his work in the hayfields of the Platte Valley. When Perry married Janet, his wife of fourteen years, he began his career in computers. He and his family now reside in Shawnee, Kansas, a suburb of Kansas City. Co-founder of a computer consulting firm, System Solutions (www.syssolutions.com), he relaxes by helping with youth wrestling, soccer, and baseball; cheering for the Nebraska Cornhuskers; and playing ,especially DADsercise, with his three children.

www.ingramcontent.com/pod-product-compliance
Lightning Source LLC
Chambersburg PA
CBHW031251280526
45784CB00004B/1810